THE
EVERYTHING.
GUIDE TO
PREVENTING HEART DISEASE

Dear Reader,

Through years working in the emergency department, I saw the devastation caused by heart attacks and strokes. I did not want that to be my fate or the fate of those I cared about. As an emergency physician, though, I too often see patients when it is too late.

I have spent years studying and performing research on cardiovascular disease. Wanting to reduce my own chances of early disease and disability, I have implemented the lifestyle changes that can help prevent heart disease. Through years of study and practice, I have learned the challenges to making it work in our daily lives. I did not want to just talk the talk, so that we can all walk the walk.

The greatest treatment for heart disease is prevention. Therefore, my purpose in writing this book is so that I will never see you in my emergency room.

Yours in living while enjoying life,

Murdoc Khaleghi, MD

Welcome to the EVERYTHING® Series!

These handy, accessible books give you all you need to tackle a difficult project, gain a new hobby, comprehend a fascinating topic, prepare for an exam, or even brush up on something you learned back in school but have since forgotten.

You can choose to read an Everything® book from cover to cover or just pick out the information you want from our four useful boxes: e-questions, e-facts, e-alerts, and e-ssentials.

We give you everything you need to know on the subject, but throw in a lot of fun stuff along the way, too.

We now have more than 400 Everything® books in print, spanning such wide-ranging categories as weddings, pregnancy, cooking, music instruction, foreign language, crafts, pets, New Age, and so much more. When you're done reading them all, you can finally say you know Everything®!

QUESTION

Answers to
common questions

FACT

Important snippets
of information

ALERT

Urgent
warnings

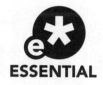

ESSENTIAL

Quick
handy tips

PUBLISHER Karen Cooper

DIRECTOR OF ACQUISITIONS AND INNOVATION Paula Munier

MANAGING EDITOR, EVERYTHING® SERIES Lisa Laing

COPY CHIEF Casey Ebert

ASSISTANT PRODUCTION EDITOR Jacob Erickson

ACQUISITIONS EDITOR Kate Powers

ASSOCIATE DEVELOPMENT EDITOR Hillary Thompson

EDITORIAL ASSISTANT Ross Weisman

EVERYTHING® SERIES COVER DESIGNER Erin Alexander

LAYOUT DESIGNERS Colleen Cunningham, Elisabeth Lariviere, Ashley Vierra, Denise Wallace

Visit the entire Everything® series at *www.everything.com*

THE
EVERYTHING®
GUIDE TO
PREVENTING
HEART DISEASE

All you need to know to
lower your blood pressure, beat high cholesterol,
and stop heart disease in its tracks

Murdoc Khaleghi, MD

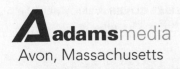
Avon, Massachusetts

This book is dedicated to all my patients who
taught me long before I could teach anyone.

An Everything® Series Book.
Everything® and everything.com® are registered trademarks of F+W Media, Inc.

Published by Adams Media, a division of F+W Media, Inc.
57 Littlefield Street, Avon, MA 02322 U.S.A.
www.adamsmedia.com

The Everything® Guide to Preventing Heart Disease contains material adapted and abridged from: *The Everything® Low Cholesterol Cookbook*, by Linda Larsen, copyright © 2007 by F+W Media, Inc., ISBN 10: 1-59869-401-4; ISBN 13: 978-1-59869-401-7; *The Everything® Low-Salt Cookbook*, by Pamela Rice Hahn, copyright © 2004 by F+W Media, Inc., ISBN 10: 1-59337-044-X; ISBN 13: 978-1-59337-044-2; *The Everything® Low Cholesterol Book, 2nd Edition*, by Murdoc Khaleghi, copyright © 2010, 2005 by F+W Media, Inc., ISBN 10: 1-4405-0551-9; ISBN 13: 978-1-4405-0551-5; *The Everything® Guide to Stress Management*, by Melissa Roberts, copyright © 2011 by F+W Media, Inc., ISBN 10: 1-4405-1087-3; ISBN 13: 978-1-4405-1087-8; and *The Everything® Guide to Meditation for Healthy Living with CD*, by David B. Dillard-Wright, PhD and Ravinder Jerath, MD, copyright © 2011 by F+W Media, Inc., ISBN 10: 1-4405-1088-1; ISBN 13: 978-1-4405-1088-5.

ISBN 10: 1-4405-2820-9
ISBN 13: 978-1-4405-2820-0
eISBN 10: 1-4405-2888-8
eISBN 13: 978-1-4405-2888-0

Printed in the United States of America.

10 9 8 7 6 5 4 3 2 1

Library of Congress Cataloging-in-Publication Data
is available from the publisher.

The information in this book should not be used for diagnosing or treating any health problem. Not all diet and exercise plans suit everyone. You should always consult a trained medical professional before starting a diet, taking any form of medication, or embarking on any fitness or weight-training program. The author and publisher disclaim any liability arising directly or indirectly from the use of this book.

Many of the designations used by manufacturers and sellers to distinguish their products are claimed as trademarks. Where those designations appear in this book and Adams Media was aware of a trademark claim, the designations have been printed with initial capital letters.

This book is available at quantity discounts for bulk purchases.
For information, please call 1-800-289-0963.

Contents

Acknowledgments

I want to thank my fantastic literary agent, Neil Salkind, and the person who reached out to me to write this book, Kate Powers at Adams Media, for helping me help others. Thanks to my colleagues and friends at EmCare, Westfield Emergency Physicians, and Holyoke and Noble Hospitals for encouraging all my pursuits. My research and studies would never have been possible without the generous opportunities at the University of California, San Diego College and Medical School, including numerous scholarships and fellowships.

Thank you to Andy, Alyssa, and PJ, who have allowed me to write another book in between games of "Apples to Apples" and watching *Wipeout*. Finally, thank you to Laura, for just everything.

The Top 10 Things You Need to Know about Heart Disease

1. Heart disease can cause severe disability and death.

2. *Anyone* can have heart disease.

3. There is no way to know if you are at risk for heart disease without getting checked for risk factors such as diabetes, high cholesterol, and high blood pressure.

4. Getting checked for risk factors is simple and does not cost a lot.

5. For many cardiovascular diseases, the most effective treatment is prevention.

6. No matter your background, you can significantly reduce your chances of early death and disability from heart disease.

7. Lifestyle changes are generally as or more effective at preventing heart disease than medications.

8. Being active at least thirty minutes several times per week, not smoking, and reducing stress can help prevent heart disease.

9. Eating fewer calories, saturated fats, and trans fats and consuming more complex carbohydrates and fiber are key to modifying risk factors.

10. The lifestyle changes that prevent heart disease do so by various means such as decreasing high blood pressure, high blood sugar, and cholesterol. Therefore, changing your lifestyle can save your life.

Introduction

YOU MAY HAVE HEARD of heart disease. Every day it seems a new article comes out about what heart disease does or what affects your heart. Not many people, though, know the full story.

Heart disease is known to be associated with heart attacks, strokes, and other cardiovascular diseases. High blood pressure, high cholesterol, and diabetes may put you at risk. By understanding and managing these risk factors, you can avoid premature death and disability.

Having these risk factors causes buildup in your arteries, the blood vessels that deliver oxygen and nutrients to your brain. When these arteries get too clogged, parts of your organs cannot receive what cells need to survive. If this happens in the blood vessels to the heart, you may develop a heart attack. If this happens in the blood vessels to your brain, you would suffer a stroke. These diseases can leave you disabled, paralyzed, or even kill you.

What you might not know is that you can modify your risk factors and decrease the chance that you will ever develop heart disease. If you know how to lower the bad type of cholesterol and increase the good type, you can significantly prevent clogging or even unclog your arteries, reducing your chance of suffering heart attacks and strokes.

To start to manage your risk factors, you need to get tested beginning at a fairly young age. These tests require repeating every few years, and if you are at higher risk, you may need testing more often to determine the proper treatment. This knowledge will help to guide you as you implement changes in your life to improve what puts you at risk.

Heart disease can be greatly influenced by your diet, physical activity, if you smoke, your weight, and your levels of stress. By making certain changes in these areas, you can reduce your chance of early death and disability. Simple changes, such as eating fewer calories and bad fats in exchange for more fiber, nutrients, and good fats, can tremendously influence your risk of heart disease. Even a modest amount of physical activity a few days a week, no matter what the activity, can have a huge impact. Not smoking and reducing stress can also make a significant impact on your risk.

These changes work by modifying many risk factors at once, such as lowering your blood pressure, cholesterol, and blood sugar. Also, such changes in your lifestyle will give you more energy and an improved mood, enriching the quality of your life.

Over the past twenty years, significant progress has been made in developing medications that address diabetes, high blood pressure, and high cholesterol and reduce the chance of cardiovascular disease. These medications can create negative side effects, but the benefits may outweigh the risks.

Overall, by understanding heart disease, how it acts, what you can do to manage it, and how to implement those actions, you can influence your future health tremendously, while potentially improving your current life.

CHAPTER 1

Heart Disease

In an instant, heart disease can tear a family apart. Abruptly, it can sever ties among spouses, parents and children, friends, neighbors, and other loved ones. Imagine how the sudden death or paralysis of you or a loved one would affect every aspect of your life. The good news in this grim scenario is that with knowledge and action, you can take significant steps toward reducing the heavy toll from this disease. Understanding what heart disease is and what contributes to it is an important first step.

What Is Heart Disease?

A healthy heart and well-functioning circulatory system are things that many people take for granted—that is, until one day they experience chest pains or breathlessness and realize that something in the body is no longer working the way it should. But what keeps a heart healthy? Or, what causes a heart to lose its ability to function properly?

The Structure and Function of the Heart

Before you can clearly understand what is going on when the heart does not work correctly, you should have a basic comprehension of its optimal structure and function. The human heart lies in the upper left center of the chest, next to the lungs. Blood flows into the right side of the heart and out of the left side. To guide the flow of blood in one constant direction, each chamber connects to the next one through valves that open when the heart contracts.

Deoxygenated blood that no longer contains as much oxygen, because the oxygen has been used by the organs, enters the right side of the heart through a large vein called the vena cava. From the right ventricle, the blood enters the pulmonary artery to reacquire oxygen in the lungs. The newly oxygen-rich blood leaves the lungs and flows back to the heart's left side. When this section contracts, blood then rushes into the aorta to repeat its journey around the body. When blood reaches all the organs, it releases oxygen for the body to use to make energy. Once the blood gives up this oxygen, it returns to the heart. This circulatory process continues automatically for as long as you live, and your life is dependent on it.

FACT

The circulatory system includes the heart, lungs, and all of the blood vessels. In the average person, these vessels would be 100,000 miles long if laid end to end. The heart pumps blood through these vessels to deliver oxygen and nutrients throughout the body and to remove carbon dioxide and other cellular waste products.

When you are reclining on a couch in a primarily horizontal position, your heart does not have to work as hard to circulate blood around your body, since it does not have to flow against gravity. When you stand up from the couch—let's say to get a drink from the refrigerator—your heart must work harder to pump blood against gravity and to your working muscles. If you choose to play a sport or go for a run, often the heart has to work extra hard to meet the demands of your muscles that are quickly using oxygen. In a person with a healthy heart, all of these adaptations occur effortlessly. Many never pause to think about how their movements increase the demands on their circulatory system; they simply go, and assume that their body will respond smoothly and easily.

The function of the heart and the circulatory system is to keep blood flowing continuously at a consistent rate. This ensures delivery of essential oxygen and nutrients to the body's tissues. Other processes that occur simultaneously through the circulation include the removal of waste products from cells back to the lungs, liver, and kidneys for filtering. A healthy nervous system is also important to a healthy circulatory system, since it affects heart rate and vessel function.

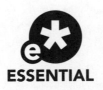

ESSENTIAL

A healthy heart is an electronically regulated muscular pump that is about the size of a fist. Each day and night, the average heart beats approximately 100,000 times and pumps 2,000 gallons of blood. Over a normal life span, the heart will beat more than 2.5 billion times.

What Can Go Wrong with the Heart?

Unfortunately, the heart doesn't always function perfectly. To comprehend the processes of atherosclerosis and their impact on heart diseases, you need to be able to understand them in the context of the range of potential heart problems. There are several disorders that can have a negative effect on the circulatory process by reducing blood flow. The most common disorders are:

- Arrhythmias or malfunctions of the electrical system, causing an irregular heartbeat
- Congestive heart failure or weakness of the muscular pump, causing fluid to back up into the lungs and other organs

- Congenital defects such as a hole between the two atrial chambers (an atrial septal defect)
- Narrowing of the heart valves from calcification (stenosis) or from tumors in the heart
- Leaking valves, known as insufficiency, so the blood does not flow through chambers optimally
- Damage to the heart muscle itself from blockage of coronary arteries due to atherosclerosis

Each of these disorders results in a heart muscle that is not capable of pumping blood sufficiently. All of these, with the exception of congenital defects, can be caused by heart attacks. The principal cause of coronary artery disease is atherosclerosis, or hardening of the arteries. Atherosclerosis comes from the root words "atheroma" and "sclerosis," which means "to harden." Atherosclerosis is a process that leads to a group of diseases characterized by the thickening of artery walls. The thickening results from a buildup of plaque on the arterial walls made up of various types of debris that collect on areas of inflammation on blood vessel walls, causing more and more narrowing of the passage through which blood can flow.

The Process Can Be Fast or Slow

The clots that block blood flow to your heart may come on slowly or quickly. The slow process, atherosclerosis, is the progressive buildup of plaque within blood vessels. Pathways become smaller and smaller, until not enough blood will flow through the vessel to meet the demand. The process is quick when plaque breaks in one blood vessel and travels to a smaller vessel, where it is trapped and stops all blood flow. This is an embolism. The two processes can also work together; atherosclerosis thins the vessel and plaque gets stuck in the thinner vessel.

What Is a Heart Attack?

When plaque in a blood vessel that feeds the heart breaks off and completely blocks the flow of blood and oxygen, a heart attack occurs. The heart, like any other part of your body, requires oxygen to survive. Without oxygen, heart tissue begins to die. This is a heart attack.

What Causes the Plaques to Grow and Break?

Plaque is formed in a variety of shapes and sizes. Small plaques accumulate throughout the arteries in the entire body and can be difficult to detect. Doctors can more easily discover the large, hardened plaques in the coronary arteries. Small plaque buildups, however, are just as concerning as thick, hard plaques. Researchers have determined that these smaller plaques are less solid on the outside and, consequently, less stable. If a small plaque buildup in the coronary arteries ruptures and forms a blood clot, it can trigger a heart attack. As a plaque then travels down a blood vessel, a smaller part of the blood vessel or more plaque may also tighten the pathway.

Plaques form for several reasons. Certain types of cholesterol deposit fat along blood vessels. Interestingly, other types of cholesterol can actually carry plaque away. When your blood pressure is high, plaque is pushed along the sides of blood vessels. Also, those blood vessels thicken, having to fight against the higher blood pressure, which strengthens the vessels against the blood pressure, but also further narrows the pathway for blood and makes it easier for plaque to get blocked should it break off. Many other risk factors and activities can affect plaque growth and blood vessel size directly and indirectly, such as genes, gender, smoking, exercise, stress, and obesity.

What Can Happen During a Heart Attack?

The range of symptoms during a heart attack can vary widely from nothing at all to death. As discussed, a heart attack occurs when heart cells begin to die from a lack of flow of oxygen-carrying blood. The symptoms depend on what heart cells die and how much. Most of the time, when heart cells begin to die, people experience pain in the chest. This does not mean that all chest pain is a heart attack, nor do all people who have heart attacks have chest pain, but in general, chest pain remains the most common and well known symptom of a heart attack.

Chest pain occurs because the nerves feeding the heart are also the nerves that feed the chest, so when heart cells begin to die, that pain is felt in the chest. The pain is most typically in the center of the chest where the nerves feed, as opposed to the left side of the chest where the heart sits. The irritation of these nerves may also cause shortness of breath, nausea, sweating, and dizziness/lightheadedness. These other symptoms may occur without chest pain. The variety of what symptoms may occur represent a great challenge to knowing when a heart attack may be occurring. Of even greater challenge is the fact that heart attacks may occur without any symptoms at all. These are also known as a "silent" heart attack, and while they can occur in anyone, are more common in women, the elderly, and diabetics.

The Effects of a Heart Attack

The residual effects of a heart attack depend on how much and what type of heart cells die. Your heart, like many other parts of your body, has a certain amount of "reserve capacity." This means that even if some of your heart cells die, your heart can often still perform 100 percent of its function. This is why if you suspect a heart attack, it is important to immediately seek medical care. Oftentimes, medical or procedural intervention can help restore blood flow to the heart and therefore minimize the number of heart cells that die and the impact of the heart attack on the body.

Should too many heart cells die, the heart can no longer pump most effectively. The weakened heart has a more difficult time pumping blood to all the tissues of the body; those tissues do not effectively receive all the essential nutrients contained in blood, hurting your body's function and its ability to heal. In addition, because blood is not pumped as effectively away from the lungs, fluid can back up into the lungs, potentially causing difficulty breathing. Fluid can further back up from the lungs into the rest of the body, causing symptoms like liver and leg swelling. Overall, this backup of fluid from the heart is known as congestive heart failure or CHF, as the failure of the heart causes congestion in other parts of the body.

Should the heart cells that die be certain cells in the heart's pacemaker, the heart can develop an arrhythmia, or disturbance in the rhythm of the heart. The arrhythmia can vary from the heart beating fast, slow, or irregularly. What can make heart attacks immediately deadly is if the disturbance in heart rhythm is so significant that the heart can no longer beat in a way that pumps blood to the rest of the body. Such a disturbance in heart function can cause death within minutes. It's for this reason that there's a growing prevalence of automatic external defibrillators or AEDs in public areas. A shock from an AED can potentially resynchronize the electricity in the heart's pacemaker to restore effective pumping.

Is the Heart the Only Thing Worth Caring About?

While heart disease is the leading killer of men and women, the process that causes heart disease causes many other serious diseases that can also cause severe disability and death.

Cardiovascular Disease

The two biggest killers, strokes and heart disease, come in a variety of life-threatening forms. All these diseases are referred to as cardiovascular diseases (CVDs). CVDs also include high blood pressure, coronary heart disease, congestive heart failure, stroke, rheumatic heart disease, artery diseases, pulmonary heart disease, and congenital cardiovascular defects. Artheroembolic disease of the arteries that supply the heart is known as coronary heart disease or coronary artery disease (CAD).

It is possible for a person to have more than one type of cardiovascular disease at the same time. In fact, many people have multiple cardiovascular disorders at once, as having one cardiovascular disorder increases the risk for having another. For example, a person may have both coronary artery disease and high blood pressure. Coronary artery disease is responsible for more than half of all heart attacks in men and women under age seventy-five.

ESSENTIAL

According to government statistics, if all forms of major cardiovascular disease (CVD) were eliminated, life expectancy would rise by almost seven years. Compared with that, if all forms of cancer were eliminated, the gain would be only three years. The probability at birth of eventually dying from major CVD is almost 50 percent, while the chance of dying from cancer is approximately 22 percent.

Scientists now know that atherosclerosis can start in childhood. Researchers have found the beginning of fatty streaks in the arteries of children as young as three years old. The average American has significant buildup in his arterial walls by middle age. In women, possibly because of the protective effects of estrogen, the thicker buildups do not begin to show up until after menopause.

Even without the impact of a stroke or heart attack, atherosclerosis advances the aging process. Healthy circulation in the body is the source of nutrition and life for the cells. As this circulation is slowly cut off, it impairs the functioning of your cells. Atherosclerosis does not need to be inevitable. With knowledge of the mechanisms that contribute to this disease, you can take steps to reduce your risks and to prolong your youthful vitality and energy.

Atherosclerosis and Coronary Artery Disease

The principal cause of coronary artery disease is atherosclerosis or hardening of the arteries. Remember, most people with cardiovascular disease will not have advance notice that reveals deadly plaques before they happen. To avoid the two most common and deadliest diseases, you must act even before the warning signs, because often by the time you get warning signs it may be too late. By understanding the nature of cardiovascular disease and what can be done to prevent it, only then can you act to prevent early death or disability.

Through effective management of what puts you at risk, you can cut your risks of having a future heart attack and add years to your life. At the same time, beyond extending your longevity, improving your lifestyle habits can also enrich the quality of those additional years of living. It is possible to become even healthier as you age; suffering years of disease, disability, and loss of vitality is not anyone's necessary fate. By working to improve your health, you can add years to your life and get even more enjoyment out of life. You can also save thousands of dollars in medical bills and perhaps far more in productivity.

What Is a Stroke or Brain Attack?

The brain needs oxygen to survive, like the heart and every other part of the body. It obtains that oxygen from blood that is transported through the blood vessels. Any obstruction to that blood flow will cause the brain to die. And just as every part of your body is dependent on the heart, it is also dependent on the brain. The brain controls all aspects of thinking, movement, and sensation, and if it stops working, everything else will, too. A stroke is essentially a "brain attack."

How Do You Have a Stroke?

Both atherosclerosis and embolisms may obstruct blood flow to the brain and cause the dysfunction of some parts or nearly all of the brain. Strokes are just as devastating to people and families as heart attacks, and in some ways can be even more devastating.

Strokes can cause permanent damage that affects every aspect of basic neurologic functioning. They can paralyze, making the victim unable to use a certain extremity or side of the body. They can affect thinking, so that the victim cannot speak with the right words. They can also affect understanding—many sufferers are not able to comprehend what is in front of them. Strokes can steal away the ability to remember the most basic things. They can even affect swallowing, forcing patients to eat through a tube inserted directly in the stomach. A severe stroke can result in extreme disability or death. According to the Centers for Disease Control and Prevention, when considered separately from other cardiovascular diseases, stroke is the third-leading cause of death in the United States.

ALERT

If you feel that someone may have suffered a stroke or heart attack, get the victim to a hospital as soon as possible. Be sure to call the hospital and let it know you are on the way or, even better, call 911 and wait for the ambulance.

How Do You Treat a Stroke?

While there are still certain treatments for strokes, they are far less expansive and effective than the multitude of heart attack treatments that have developed over the last decade. Unless the stroke is treated within several hours of onset, most of what doctors can do is just watchful waiting to see whether the stroke results in disability. Further tests and treatments are only potentially able to prevent future strokes. Even within the first few hours, the treatments are often ineffective. Since treatment options are minimal once someone has a stroke, the main method of combating strokes is trying to prevent them from ever occurring. Prevention is also the best way to fight heart attacks and other cardiovascular disease.

FACT

According to the American Heart Association and American Stroke Association, approximately 40,000 more women than men have strokes annually. Experts believe that this is because women tend to live longer than men, and the highest rates for stroke are among those in the oldest age groups.

A mild or mini-stroke, described as a transient ischemic attack (TIA), can end in a matter of minutes. The damage can include mild weakness or numbness in an arm or a leg or slight difficulty with speech. This can be a warning sign of a larger impending stroke.

Can Anywhere Else Be Attacked?

Atherosclerosis not only affects the arteries that supply blood to the heart and to the brain, it can also affect the vessels that supply blood to the other parts of the body, including legs, intestines, and even erectile tissues.

Peripheral Arterial Disease

When blood flow is blocked to the legs, this condition is known as peripheral arterial disease (PAD). Clogging of these arteries leads to discomfort in the legs that can become more severe as time goes on. You are much more likely to have a heart attack or stroke if you have this condition.

Warning signs and symptoms of PAD include:

- Cramping, heaviness, fatigue, or aching of the buttocks, thighs, or calves when walking

- Leg pain that occurs when you walk uphill, carry heavy loads, or walk quickly
- Aching of the foot that worsens at night and is relieved by standing up or by allowing the foot to hang off the edge of the bed
- Leg pain that stops when you stand still or rest

If allowed to progress, peripheral artery disease can lead to lack of blood flow to the feet. The feet, like any other body part, cannot survive without blood flow. If not corrected in time, the only treatment is amputation.

Erectile Dysfunction and Intestinal Atherosclerosis

Erectile dysfunction or impotence is often associated with atherosclerotic plaque buildup. According to the National Institute of Diabetes and Digestive and Kidney Diseases, about 5 percent of forty-year-old men and 15–25 percent of sixty-five-year-old men experience erectile dysfunction. In addition, when smoking is part of the picture, the odds of erectile dysfunction increase even further. Male smokers have approximately a 30 percent higher risk for erectile dysfunction when compared with nonsmokers. However, just as hardening of the arteries is not inevitable with aging, neither is the loss of potency. Maintaining health of the heart and circulatory system can also help maintain this aspect of youthful vigor and vitality.

FACT

Erectile dysfunction affects 15–30 million American men, depending on exactly how it is defined. Approximately 70 percent of all cases are due to diseases such as atherosclerosis, vascular disease, diabetes, kidney disease, multiple sclerosis, neurological disease, and chronic alcoholism.

Even the intestines' blood flow can become blocked, causing intense stomach pains. Sadly, this disease is incredibly hard to diagnose, as there are so many other causes of stomach pain. By the time an intestinal stroke is discovered, death is the usual outcome. Once again, the best method of treating this disease is avoidance through prevention.

Factors That Put You at Risk

You are not completely in control of whether you will develop heart disease. At the same time, however, you are far from being totally helpless. There are many steps you can take to lessen your risk of developing heart disease. But before you can reduce your risks and improve your odds, you need to know what those risks are.

Leading Risk Factors

Multiple factors contribute to the development and progression of heart disease, and the more factors you possess the greater your likelihood of having it. One risky characteristic alone, such as your age, may be enough to trigger the disease. However, a combination of factors, such as age, inactivity, smoking, and improper nutrition, will put you at much higher risk for heart attacks and strokes.

FACT

To determine your risk score according to the information gathered by the Framingham Study, use the online calculator at *http://hp2010 .nhlbihin.net/atpiii/calculator.asp?usertype=prof*. Keep in mind that subjects in this study were primarily Caucasian, middle aged, and without heart disease. It may not be completely accurate for other groups, but it is still useful as a general guide.

The leading risk factors for heart disease are:

- High LDL cholesterol
- Low HDL cholesterol
- Diabetes
- Cigarette smoking or inhaling secondary smoke
- Hypertension or high blood pressure
- Unmanaged stress
- Physical inactivity or a sedentary lifestyle
- Excess weight

- Family history of heart disease
- Age and gender

Any condition that indicates the presence of atherosclerosis also indicates a high risk of coronary artery disease. In other words, having a stroke puts you at higher risk for a heart attack.

Risk Factors That Cannot Be Changed

While some risk factors for heart disease cannot be changed, it is important to know the best way to influence those factors. Treating and or keeping an eye on one risk factor often affects others, thereby reducing your overall chances of developing cardiovascular disease.

Family History

Family history is an important consideration when determining your risk for heart disease. If you have a first-degree female relative (mother, sister, or daughter) under the age of sixty-five or a first-degree male relative (father, brother, son) under fifty-five who has heart disease, that is a risk factor for you. If your parents have heart disease, then you are more likely to develop it. No one can change his genes, but if you have a family history of heart disease, it is even more important for you to assess your risk factors and to have annual checkups.

Your Age and Gender

Men are at a greater risk than women of developing heart disease in middle age. From the age of forty-five, a man's risk of heart disease increases, and this risk continues to increase with age. By the age of sixty-five, half of all American men are likely to have coronary artery disease.

Women enjoy some protection from heart disease that may come from the hormone estrogen. Women who are fifty-five years of age and older, however, are at an increased risk of heart disease. Hormone replacement therapy has not been shown to reduce this risk. As with men, this risk continues to increase with age. By the age of sixty-five, a third of all American women are likely to have coronary artery disease.

CHAPTER 2

Blood Pressure

Perhaps the most long-standing and well-known risk factor for heart disease is high blood pressure, otherwise known as hypertension. Over the last several decades, physicians have been more aggressively treating high blood pressure in the hopes of reducing the long-term incidence of cardio-vascular disease. To understand how to modify high blood pressure, it is important to understand what is.

What Is Blood Pressure?

Pressure equals the force of something over a certain area. In the case of the blood pressure, the force is exerted by blood vessels on vessel walls. In response to such pressure, blood vessel walls must mold and strengthen themselves to be able to withstand such pressure and assure that an appropriate amount of blood is pumped to your organs.

Blood Pressure Basics

Blood pressure has two values, shown as an upper number and a lower number. The upper number represents the systolic blood pressure, or the greater pressure exerted by the heart and blood when the heart is pumping. The lower number or diastolic pressure represents the pressure of the blood when the heart is relaxed.

The pressure is measured in millimeters of mercury, also written as mmHg. Normally, the systolic blood pressure ranges from 90mmHg–120mmHg, and the diastolic blood pressure is less than 80mmHg. Blood pressure can vary significantly depending on time of day, activity, emotions, recent meal, and many other factors.

Low Blood Pressure

While most attention is given to high blood pressure, as it's one of the leading risk factors for heart disease over a long period of time, low blood pressure can be quite dangerous; in fact, the danger of low blood pressure is far more immediate. If blood pressure is low, that means organs are not receiving an adequate amount of blood. This can cause symptoms such as lightheadedness, especially when standing, from not enough blood going to the brain. One of the causes of low blood pressure may be that the heart is not pumping blood effectively, due to congestive heart failure or an arrhythmia due to a heart attack. Excessively treating high blood pressure can also result in low blood pressure. The danger of low blood pressure does not take away from your need to address high blood pressure, though it does highlight dangerous side effects—a careful balance must be struck.

Why Does Blood Pressure Get High?

You are not born with high blood pressure; something happens in your life to get it that way. Different people have high blood pressure for different reasons, but if you understand the major contributors to high blood pressure, you can then attempt to address those causes.

You Are What You Eat

As we delve further in this book, you will learn more about how what you eat can significantly affect atherosclerosis and your long-term blood pressure. Blood pressure can be affected far more immediately, though, by your salt intake. The most common form of salt is sodium chloride. The amount of sodium you ingest significantly affects your blood pressure on a day-to-day basis. The reason for this is osmosis.

Osmosis is the general scientific concept that fluid tends to travel from where there's a higher concentration of fluid to where there is a lower concentration. When you ingest salt, because there is now a higher concentration of salt in your body, there is a lower concentration of fluid. In an attempt to normalize this concentration of fluid, your body holds onto more fluid. As you have learned, though, blood pressure is pressure exerted by the blood in your body on vessel walls. If there's more fluid in the blood, the pressure exerted on those walls is higher, giving you higher blood pressure. In other words, eating salt can immediately raise your blood pressure.

FACT

Though high blood pressure is often investigated to find a potential medical cause, over 90 percent of cases of high blood pressure are called "essential hypertension," where no medical cause has been found.

While it's true that having elevated blood pressure for just one day, week, or even longer may not be that serious in terms of the long-term affect on your health, most people who eat extra salt tend to do it often for most of their lives. In other words, the chronic ingestion of salt can chronically raise your blood pressure.

Stress and Blood Pressure

For years people have said to watch your stress or you will raise your blood pressure. This old wives' tale has been confirmed over years of research, and makes sense if you examine how our bodies are designed. Over millions of years, the human body developed a stress response. This response emerged in situations such as being chased by a vicious animal. In this fight-or-flight response, your heart pumps harder and your blood vessels tighten to get more blood to your muscles so you can run faster. These changes elevate your blood pressure.

In addition, your body breaks down more of your stored blood sugar, increasing the level of blood sugar in your body, so that you have more fuel for your harder working tissues as well. This elevated blood sugar contributes to long-term heart disease as well. So while these short-term stress responses may benefit us, the long-term chronic stress that many live under contributes to heart disease in many ways.

Blood Pressure and Aging

Over years, many factors contribute to increasing blood pressure as you age. Your blood vessels become harder as you age. A part of this hardening is the normal process of aging. Also, blood vessels can thicken in response to high blood pressure, which can then contribute to high blood pressure. This shows the significant benefit of early prevention; early modification of blood pressure can benefit not just short-term blood pressure, but long-term blood pressure, as well. Atherosclerosis, the process of plaque formation, also hardens blood vessels.

ALERT

Some cases of high blood pressure are caused by hormonal disorders. Usually these show other signs as well. Even without other signs, testing is done in those who develop high blood pressure at a very young age, because their blood pressure usually remains high despite lifestyle adjustment and medications.

Since many risk factors influence the hardening of blood vessels, modifying certain risk factors for heart disease can decrease other risk factors as well. For example, healthful eating, regular exercise, and not smoking can reduce atherosclerosis and therefore help prevent heart disease. By decreasing the hardening of blood vessels, such lifestyle habits improve blood pressure. In fact, these lifestyle habits have also been shown to improve blood pressure in other ways. Once you understand risk factors, you can then understand that the same lifestyle habits influence all risk factors; therefore, focusing on certain lifestyle modifications will give you the most benefit.

High Blood Pressure and Your Heart

You know that high blood pressure is a risk factor for heart disease, but how? Over years, due to aging and certain unhealthy lifestyle habits, blood pressures tend to increase. Such an increase affects many parts your body, with these affects then increasing your chance for heart disease.

Your Blood Vessels

When blood pressure is elevated, the walls of your blood vessels become thickened and less elastic. This thickening makes it harder for blood to flow through your vessels, and the decrease in elasticity causes greater damage to the vessel walls. Such damage causes plaques to form, a major contributor to heart attacks and strokes. Over time this thickening and loss of elasticity further decreases the ability of blood vessels to relax and respond appropriately to your body's hormonal signals. The inability of blood vessels to relax further increases blood pressure, and the cycle continues. The connectedness of your blood vessels and heart is so strong that you really can't think of disease in either one in isolation. This is why, instead of heart disease, the more appropriate term is cardiovascular disease, referring to both your heart (cardio) and your blood vessels (vascular). This connectedness also reveals why heart disease is linked to so many other forms of vascular disease, such as strokes and peripheral vascular disease. If your heart is disturbed, it's likely the body's blood vessels are as well, and vice-versa, which puts many other organs at risk.

Your Heart

The increased pressure also means the heart has to pump blood with a greater force. When the heart has to pump harder, it remodels itself to be able to pump with greater strength. Though certain types of remodeling of the heart can be healthy—such as the remodeling athletes' hearts undergo as they build muscle to accommodate exercise—this type can be dangerous. As the heart builds more muscle to pump against the higher blood pressure, the heart muscle thickens. The heart may thicken so much that it actually becomes difficult for blood to flow into the heart, leading to the backup of fluid into the lungs or congestive heart failure.

In addition, the greater demand on the heart, as well as the thick muscle, means the heart requires more blood and oxygen to supply this demand. Unfortunately, many people with high blood pressure actually have atherosclerosis in the blood vessels that feed the heart. So while the heart in a person with high blood pressure may need extra blood flow, often blood is hindered by the buildup of plaque due to cardiovascular disease and the thickening of the blood vessels due to high blood pressure. In other words, there may be decreased blood flow in the hearts that need it most, and as mentioned, when there's not enough blood flow to meet the heart's demand, problems may range from the heart getting irritated by the lack of oxygen to a severe heart attack.

Your Organs

When the blood vessels feeding your organs do not function well, thereby upsetting the flow of oxygen and other nutrient-carrying blood to your organs, they cannot function properly. This may occur as a sudden change from a plaque breaking off, such as in your heart, brain, legs, or abdomen. This can also occur as a progressive dysfunction as well. For example, when kidneys are constantly exposed to higher blood pressure, they do not work as well. This is especially important in the kidneys because they have a vital role in regulating blood pressure. So when the kidney does not work as well due to problems such as high blood pressure, you may face even higher blood pressure. This higher blood pressure occurs in addition to all sorts of other medical problems that occur when kidneys do not function as well.

Once again, cardiovascular disease and its risk factors, when not dealt with and corrected, can get caught in a vicious, worsening cycle.

ALERT

High blood pressure is one of the most prevalent diseases in society, and its prevalence increases as the population ages because blood pressure gets higher as humans age. Because of its prevalence and the harm it can cause when unrecognized, decreasing high blood pressure is one of the most effective preventative measures you have for reducing cardiovascular disease.

Get to Know Your Blood Pressure

Some people do not know their blood pressure at all. Some know the number, but do not understand what it means. Still others know what the number means, but not how it impacts their lives and how they should respond. Now that you understand the importance of blood pressure, read on to learn how to use this knowledge.

The Numbers

The threshold for elevated blood pressure is 140/90 mmHg. The device to measure blood pressure is a sphygmomanometer, also known as a blood pressure cuff. Every physician or physician's office has one, and they are in nearly every pharmacy and other health care setting. Some of the devices are manual and need to be operated by someone else; others are automatic that you can use yourself. These automatic machines tend to be slightly less accurate, but are still useful.

Remember, blood pressure levels are variable, so while you are encouraged to check your blood pressure, you should not make any decisions based on a single reading. On the other hand, because your blood pressure can fluctuate so much, one of the surefire ways to elevate your blood pressure is to check it all the time, as it will occasionally be higher, causing unneeded stress in your life.

The Diagnosis

Having a systolic or diastolic blood pressure greater than these values on repeated checks will often result in a diagnosis of hypertension, but do not fear! There is much you can do to prevent high blood pressure and to correct it. Blood pressure will often respond to lifestyle changes, so that remains first-line therapy. If your blood pressure is high despite such changes, there are many medications to treat it.

ALERT

Researchers used to think that it was the diastolic, or lower blood pressure number, that mattered most to long-term health. Recent research has confirmed, though, that the systolic, diastolic, and even the pulse pressure, the difference between systolic and diastolic, all matter.

Lifestyle changes remain the method of choice for several reasons. First, they do not come with the cost and side effects of medications. In addition, lifestyle changes may affect many risk factors for heart disease, while medications usually affect only a single aspect. For example, while blood pressure medication may treat high blood pressure, it will do nothing for your cholesterol, while eating well and regular exercise can affect both. Finally, lifestyle modification not only helps prevent the sickness and death that can result from cardiovascular disease, it can also increase your quality of life, from your energy to your mood to your skin.

Early High Blood Pressure

Over the past two decades, more attention has been focused on those whose high blood pressure is in a borderline zone of above 120/90 mmHg but below the threshold for hypertension. These people, now labeled prehypertensives, often get checked more frequently and are encouraged to make lifestyle changes before becoming hypertensive. If there are multiple other cardiovascular risk factors, pharmaceutical treatment may start, as there is some benefit from escaping even this prehypertensive zone. Like with regular hypertension, all the same principles apply regarding testing, prevention, and treatment—only the threshold changes.

CHAPTER 3

Cholesterol

You don't need to be a scientist to understand what cholesterol is and how to effectively manage your levels for better health. You just need to care about your health. Cholesterol is an essential part of this life process—it keeps you going and can stop you dead in your tracks. The better you understand cholesterol, the better you can choose which of these results will occur.

What Is Cholesterol?

Cholesterol is a necessary and natural part of each and every cell in the human body and in the bodies of other animals. Cholesterol helps maintain the structure of the walls of cells and works to keep the brain healthy. The liver uses cholesterol as raw material to create important hormones and manufacture digestive enzymes. Cholesterol is integral to thinking and sexual activity as well as innumerable other bodily functions.

FACT

Most gallstones formed in the gallbladder are composed primarily of cholesterol. The liver responds to the presence of dietary fat by producing cholesterol to synthesize bile to digest the fats. If you eat too much fat, the liver may overproduce cholesterol, leading to the formation of gallstones.

A healthy liver makes cholesterol, a waxy lipid or fatlike substance. In addition, you also acquire cholesterol from the food you eat. The big picture, however, is not quite so simple; many other factors influence your cholesterol levels. Even if you are a vegetarian and don't eat foods that contain cholesterol, you will still have plenty of cholesterol in your body. Depending on the type of cholesterol and how much of each type, this can be a good or a bad thing.

Factors Affecting Cholesterol

Total cholesterol is the sum total of all the cholesterol in your bloodstream at a given time. There are different types of cholesterol, such as high-density lipoproteins (HDLs) and low-density lipoproteins (LDLs), which make up the total amount. Density refers to the weight of the lipoprotein. If cholesterol is HDL, that means it is very compact; if it is LDL, that means it is less compact and more loose. In general, HDL is good cholesterol and LDL is bad cholesterol.

Several factors affect the total cholesterol levels in your bloodstream. These factors include the following:

- **What you eat:** Foods that come from animals, such as meats and eggs, contain cholesterol that you absorb as well as saturated fats, which can convert into cholesterol in your body. Trans fats, contained in processed foods, are also converted into cholesterol.
- **Whether you are overweight:** Generally, the more fat you have the more cholesterol you have. Therefore, weight loss can often lead to cholesterol loss.
- **Whether you smoke:** Smoking both raises your cholesterol and makes the cholesterol you have more harmful.
- **Whether you consume alcohol:** For years, scientists have noticed that moderate amounts of alcohol consumption can actually help your cholesterol levels. This comes with caution, as alcohol can worsen many other aspects of your health.
- **Whether you are inactive or active regularly:** People who are physically active on a regular basis not only have better levels of cholesterol, they have more of the type that helps the body.
- **Whether you effectively manage stress in your life:** Research studies show that mental and emotional stress can raise your cholesterol and make the cholesterol you have more harmful to the body.
- **Your genes:** Your genes influence all your traits, including your cholesterol. If your parents had high cholesterol, you are more likely to have high cholesterol. In fact, there are certain common genetic disorders that will give you extremely high cholesterol, which can be incredibly harmful.
- **Your gender:** Before menopause, women have a natural advantage over men, as female hormones help maintain better cholesterol levels.
- **Age:** With time, cholesterol levels tend to worsen, causing cumulative harm, which after years can become life threatening.
- **What type of medications you take:** For certain individuals, medications can help effectively manage cholesterol levels, while other medications can actually make cholesterol worse.

You may not be able to change your age, gender, or genes, but to improve your cholesterol levels, you can certainly change how you eat, whether you smoke, and how much you exercise.

A Complicated Puzzle

Your total cholesterol levels do not paint a complete picture of the health of your arteries. Because not all cholesterol is bad, you need to find out what type of cholesterol you have. Remember that cholesterol is essential to the health of every cell in your body and to the production of your hormones. Good cholesterol, or HDL, actually helps the body function well. To fully understand the health of your arteries and what is flowing in your bloodstream, you also need to find out about the levels of other blood fats, known as triglycerides.

Half the people whose total cholesterol levels come within the desirable levels have heart disease, so simply achieving this target does not guarantee you are not at risk for heart disease. To truly evaluate your risk, you need to take into account all of the risk factors that apply to you. Pay particular attention if you have a family history of heart disease. Regardless of cholesterol levels, it is a good idea for everyone to observe healthy lifestyle habits, not only to lengthen your life but also to increase the quality of those additional years. Anyone can improve his health and reduce the risk of serious disease by improving his cholesterol.

FACT

Lipid is the chemical family name for fat. Its root is the Greek word *lipos,* meaning "fat." A blood lipid is a fat that circulates in the bloodstream. Cholesterol and triglycerides are both classified as blood lipids. A lipoprotein is a combination of fat surrounded and protected by protein to enable the fat to circulate within your mostly water-filled blood.

Separating the Good from the Bad

The major players in the cholesterol picture are the liver and the blood fats. To help the body function, the liver takes cholesterol and fat in the blood to make new cholesterol. The liver manufactures both good and bad cholesterol, manages their release into the bloodstream, and collects cholesterol back from the bloodstream. The body uses cholesterol and fat to build cell membranes, create essential hormones, and form digestive enzymes.

Lipoproteins

Fat and cholesterol need to be transported throughout the body. However, fat and cholesterol are oily and blood is watery; oil and water do not mix. This makes fat and cholesterol difficult to transport on their own. The liver resolves this transport issue by combining and coating the cholesterol with substances that are fat on one side, touching the fat and cholesterol, and protein on the other side, touching watery blood. These are called lipoproteins or combinations of fat and protein. The lipoprotein coating enables fat and cholesterol to travel in the bloodstream by shielding water-fearing fat with water-loving protein. The various types of lipoproteins are outlined in the following chart.

▼ TYPES OF LIPOPROTEINS

Name	Type of Lipoprotein	Nickname
HDL	High-density lipoprotein	"Good" cholesterol
LDL	Low-density lipoprotein	"Bad" cholesterol
VLDL	Very low-density lipoprotein	—
SDLDL	Small, dense, low-density lipoprotein	—
Lp(a)	Apolipoprotein (a) plus low-density lipoprotein	"Ugly" cholesterol

The Liver: Cholesterol Manufacturing Plant

Imagine a pickup and delivery service to and from the liver, which is the cholesterol manufacturing plant. Imagine that the lipoproteins are like delivery trucks that carry packages of cholesterol in the bloodstream. The function of the LDL delivery trucks is to package cholesterol and transport it out through the bloodstream to your various organs. Contrastingly, the function of the HDL delivery trucks is to pick up excess cholesterol packages from the bloodstream and return them to the liver for repackaging, as needed.

In a healthy body, this efficient manufacturing, pickup, and delivery system maintains perfect balance. The LDLs go out to perform their functions at the receptor stops. HDLs pick up excess LDLs that the cells don't need and deliver them back to the liver for repackaging. Trucks circulate constantly, at all hours of the day and night, providing energy for quick fuel and minimal storage reserves. The liver manufacturing plant naturally manages the entire process.

ESSENTIAL

The primary functions of the liver include metabolizing carbohydrates, proteins, and fats; storing and activating vitamins and minerals; forming and excreting bile to digest fats; converting ammonia to urea for elimination; metabolizing steroids; and acting as a filter by removing bacteria from blood. The liver also detoxifies substances such as drugs and alcohol.

HDL cholesterol, the pickup-truck fleet, is known as the "good" cholesterol. When you understand how the liver's manufacturing and transport system works, it's easy to see why the HDLs are considered good—because HDLs help transport the excess LDL cholesterol from your arteries to the liver, where it can be metabolized. Since knowing the amount of your HDL cholesterol is an important aspect of assessing your overall risk of heart disease, it's a good idea to have your HDL levels measured—not just your total cholesterol checked.

LDL cholesterol is known as the "bad" cholesterol; however, LDL cholesterol is bad for your body only if you have too much in your bloodstream or you have too much of the particularly harmful type. LDL cholesterol is an essential building block for cell membranes and the substance from which hormones, including cortisol and testosterone, are manufactured. The amount of LDL that exceeds what your body needs, however, flows through your bloodstream and increases the likelihood of the formation of plaque that can block blood flow.

Triglycerides, also referred to as TRGs, are a type of fat that circulates in your bloodstream. TRGs are composed of a sticky substance called glycerol and fatty acids. They can provide your body with a source of energy, if needed. Triglyceride levels spike immediately after you eat and decrease slowly as the body processes nutrients from food that has been consumed. If muscles are working and active, triglycerides can provide needed fuel.

If muscle cells do not use the circulating triglycerides to create energy, the TRGs are eventually deposited in the body's fat stores just like cholesterol, and just like cholesterol they can cause a clogging of your arteries.

ALERT

According to the American Heart Association, approximately 102 million Americans, or more than 50 percent of American adults, have total cholesterol levels of 200 mg/dL or higher. This level indicates increased cardiovascular risk, and for most people, this total is composed mostly of LDL cholesterol. More than half of these Americans are unaware that they have high cholesterol.

People who are overweight, who drink alcohol excessively, who are diabetic, or who have other disorders are prone to having elevated triglyceride levels. Women tend to have higher triglyceride levels than men. Evidence from research shows that the risk of heart disease increases when the triglyceride level is too high, particularly when a person simultaneously has low levels of HDL cholesterol.

Cholesterol and Your Heart

Modern living conditions overload and strain the system. By eating too much and moving too little, people make it all too easy for this delicately balanced delivery, pickup, and storage system to break down.

Breakdown of the System

The efficiency begins to fail when more LDL packages are transported in the bloodstream than are needed by the body's tissues. This excess LDL continues to circulate in the bloodstream, increasing fat levels in the bloodstream and contributing to congestion in your arteries.

If this excess LDL occurs at the same time that too few HDL trucks are available to collect and deliver it back to the liver for recycling, the LDL cholesterol starts to collect on the arterial walls. Over time, this collection of debris on the arterial walls leads to a complete blockage, which then prevents blood flow that delivers essential oxygen for survival to the body's tissues, and the body's tissues begin to die. If this happens in the muscle tissues of the heart, the result is a heart attack. If this happens in the brain, it causes a stroke. Almost any artery can get blocked, killing almost any area of your body, but the most common and important areas are your brain and heart.

The leading causes of the system breakdown are the following:

1. **Overproduction of LDL packages.** The liver produces too much LDL cholesterol for the body's needs and much more than the HDLs can pick up.
2. **Reduction of HDL pickup trucks.** The liver does not produce or release enough HDLs into the bloodstream to pick up the excess LDLs.
3. **Breakdown of liver management dispatch system.** The liver does not correctly signal to the body that it needs to pick up more LDLs.
4. **Damage to roadways.** Inflammation is present in the interior walls of the arteries.
5. **Transformation of LDL packages into litter.** Free radicals, which are breakdown products of certain bodily functions, attach to certain LDL packages and oxidize them, causing them to become large and sticky and attach to blood vessel walls.

ALERT

According to the American Heart Association, nearly 2,300 people in America die of cardiovascular disease each day, an average of one death every thirty-eight seconds. This makes cardiovascular disease the number-one killer, claiming more than one in three people.

Scientists worldwide continue to conduct research so they can thoroughly understand the roles of the different types of lipoproteins and blood fats in the mechanisms behind heart disease. Evidence from research suggests that there are many LDL and HDL subtypes. Some of these subtypes are more harmful and others are more beneficial to health. For LDL cholesterol, particle size plays a significant role in the risk picture. People with higher numbers of the small, dense LDL particles rather than the large, fluffy LDL particles have a significantly higher risk of heart attack.

The Endothelial Lining

The endothelium or endothelial lining is the tissue that lines the inside of your blood vessels, through which your nutrients travel through the bloodstream. Evidence from research studies shows that when this inner lining of the vessel walls becomes inflamed, the formation of the clogging cholesterol plaque begins. White blood cells, which fight infection, go to the inflamed area, dragging with them other substances including calcium, cholesterol, and fats. Scientists have researched how to maintain the health of the endothelial lining to prevent the initial formation of plaque.

What Is Plaque?

Plaque is composed of bad cholesterol and calcium in the bloodstream, as well as other cellular waste products that get caught in the fat deposits. As the plaque grows larger, it hardens due to the deposition of calcium. It has an outer layer of scar tissue that covers the calcium and fats as well as the white blood cells that responded to the damaged arterial wall within.

FACT

Often, heart disease is thought of as a killer in men, but it is also the number-one killer of women in America. Heart diseases kill more than half a million women each year—approximately one death per minute. The American Heart Association reports that heart diseases claim more women's lives than the next seven causes of death combined!

Eventually, the buildup of plaque can decrease or block blood flow to the heart or brain, starving these organs of essential oxygen and causing chest pains, a heart attack, or a stroke. This plaque buildup is known as atherosclerosis, and is one of the most common types of heart disease. Plaque can begin to accumulate in childhood and develops so slowly in your body that its presence often grows without any telltale signs to make you aware of it.

Get to Know Your Cholesterol

A total cholesterol level includes both forms of cholesterol: LDL, the bad cholesterol that builds up in your arteries; and HDL, the good cholesterol that collects bad cholesterol from the blood vessels. If you have a lower level of LDL cholesterol and a higher level of HDL, you reduce your likelihood for heart disease.

Breaking It Down

For a healthy heart and circulatory system, you should have HDL cholesterol levels higher than 40 mg/dL. The higher the level of your HDLs, the better it is for your health. People who have low levels of HDL cholesterol are at higher risk for heart disease.

According to the NCEP guidelines, an HDL level of 60 mg/dL is considered a negative risk factor. A negative risk factor is like a bonus point that can decrease your heart attack or stroke risk.

Since eating affects all of your levels, you should fast for at least nine to twelve hours before you have a lipid profile test, which shows your HDL, LDL, triglycerides, and all other main types of fat and cholesterol. After you undertake this nine- to twelve-hour period without eating or drinking, the levels of these fats and cholesterols circulating in your bloodstream will more accurately reflect how much of these fats are consistently present in your blood, rather than what you recently ate.

The levels for all the different types of cholesterol and fats are as follows:

▼ **NCEP CHOLESTEROL AND TRIGLYCERIDE LEVEL GUIDELINES**

Total Cholesterol Level	Category
Less than 180 mg/dL	Optimal
Less than 200 mg/dL	Desirable
200–239 mg/dL	Borderline high
240 mg/dL	High

▼ NCEP CHOLESTEROL AND TRIGLYCERIDE LEVEL GUIDELINES—continued

LDL Cholesterol Level	LDL Cholesterol Category
Less than 100 mg/dL	Optimal
100–129 mg/dL	Near optimal/above optimal
130–159 mg/dL	Borderline high
160–189 mg/dL	High
190 mg/dL and above	Very high
HDL Cholesterol Level	**HDL Cholesterol Category**
Less than 40 mg/dL	Low
60 mg/dL and above	High
Triglyceride Level	**Triglyceride Category**
Less than 150 mg/dL	Normal
150–199 mg/dL	Borderline high
200–499 mg/dL	High
500 mg/dL and above	Very high

Source: NIH Publication Nos. 01-3305 and 01-3290

CHAPTER 4

Diabetes

When you eat foods that are rich in carbohydrates, such as breads, cereals, or grains, your body breaks it down into glucose, also referred to as blood sugar. Your body can use glucose for energy. In a normally functioning system, a healthy pancreas releases insulin into the bloodstream, and this insulin helps remove the glucose from your bloodstream for your cells to use as fuel. In people who have diabetes, this process is dysfunctional. Either their bodies do not produce any insulin or the insulin they produce cannot be used.

What Is Diabetes?

Approximately 24 million Americans have diabetes; roughly one-third of these people are unaware they have it. The incidence of diabetes increases with age; about 50 percent of people with diabetes are fifty or older.

Because their bodies cannot convert the sugar in the blood into energy, people with diabetes have high levels of glucose in their bloodstream. The kidneys of diabetic people need to work extra hard to filter the blood to remove the excess glucose. This causes frequent urination and excessive thirst from fluid loss when the blood sugar is high (this happens only before the diabetes is diagnosed or when the diabetic is experiencing hyperglycemia).

The liver is also involved in the process of maintaining normal blood sugar levels. After you eat, the sugars from the food enter your bloodstream and are available as fuel, along with the triglycerides. If not all the sugar fuel is used, either due to poor processing based on low insulin or a reduced need for energy based on a low activity level, the liver removes the excess sugar from the bloodstream, much in the same manner as it removes excess cholesterol, and stores it in the liver as glycogen. If for some reason you are unable to eat, the liver can later release this stored glucose into the bloodstream to provide an energy boost. This helps keep your blood sugar levels in a more constant range.

FACT

Diabetes can lead to many dangerous conditions, particularly if untreated or incorrectly managed. These include heart disease, stroke, kidney disease and kidney failure, nerve damage, and gum disease. The disease also raises the risk threefold of dying from complications related to influenza or pneumonia. In America, diabetes is currently the sixth-leading cause of death and is a leading cause of blindness and amputations.

Diabetes consists of two main types, both characterized by the body's inability to process available sugar into energy. The two major types are type 1 and type 2 diabetes. People with either type can experience elevated blood-glucose levels or hyperglycemia.

Type 1 Diabetes

Type 1 diabetes is an autoimmune condition that occurs most often in children and adults younger than thirty. It also used to be called juvenile-onset diabetes or insulin-dependent diabetes mellitus. This condition occurs when the body does not produce any insulin, so people with this type of diabetes take daily insulin injections. Approximately 5–10 percent of people with diabetes have type 1. Young people with diabetes are not likely to have heart disease in their youth. As they age, however, their risk of heart disease is greater than those who do not have diabetes.

Type 2 Diabetes

Type 2 is the most common form of diabetes. It affects about 90–95 percent of people who have the disease. This type of diabetes used to be referred to as maturity-onset diabetes, adult-onset diabetes, or noninsulin-dependent diabetes mellitus.

Type 2 diabetes is a metabolic disorder. In this case, the pancreas produces some insulin but not enough to allow the sugar to enter the body's cells. At the same time, muscle and tissue cells develop a resistance to the insulin. Therefore, even though sugar is flowing in the bloodstream, the body's tissues remain "hungry." Scientists are still unable to identify the exact mechanism that causes insulin resistance, but it seems to have a relationship to excess body fat.

Signs and Symptoms of Diabetes

People often disregard the symptoms of diabetes. However, studies indicate that if diabetes is detected early, people can reduce the likelihood that complications will develop. Therefore, it is important to know the signs and symptoms of diabetes, particularly if you have a family history of this disease. The signs and symptoms include:

- Frequent urination
- Excessive thirst
- Extreme hunger
- Unusual weight loss
- Increased fatigue

- Irritability
- Numbness or tingling in feet or legs
- Slow-healing cuts or bruises
- Blurry vision

Diabetes and Your Heart

When a person has diabetes, she is also more likely to develop heart disease. Depending on the diabetic's number of risk factors, she may face an even greater risk of heart disease. For example, someone who has diabetes, high blood pressure, high cholesterol, who smokes, and who is completely inactive is at far greater risk of heart disease than someone who only has diabetes. Therefore, controlling risk factors that you can change is extremely important to improve overall health.

How It Works

Scientists believe that diabetes increases your risk of heart disease because persistent elevated levels of blood sugar damage arteries. If you recall how atherosclerotic plaque gets started, you will remember that plaque begins to form on areas where the inside lining of the blood vessels is damaged.

Like high blood pressure, diabetes can also cause weakness directly in the heart, known as diabetic cardiomyopathy. This weakness causes the heart to pump poorly and fluid to back up in the lungs and body (congestive heart failure). Like with high blood pressure, it can also make the heart require more blood flow, and people with risk factors such as diabetes often have less blood flow through their blood vessels.

ESSENTIAL

Diabetes increases a woman's risk of heart disease by three to seven times, compared with a twofold to threefold increase in risk for men, according to the American Heart Association. While it is important for all people with diabetes to take extra good care of their health, this is even more necessary for women.

Scientists continue to research other mechanisms to explain why people with diabetes are at such an increased risk of heart disease. Though the causality is still under debate, the fact that diabetes significantly increases your risk for heart disease is well researched and proven.

Risk and Treatment

People with diabetes have a much higher risk for heart attack and stroke. In fact, according to the American Diabetes Association, two out of every three people with diabetes will die of a heart attack or stroke. Diabetes alone raises your risk of cardiovascular disease by two to four times. In the presence of other risk factors, this number is much higher.

Fortunately, aggressive treatment of diabetes has been shown to reduce this risk significantly. Unfortunately, it's challenging for even the most compliant diabetics to maintain normal blood sugar levels all the time. The treatment of diabetes often involves injecting insulin at certain times of day. No matter how hard you work, it's pretty much impossible to be able to mimic the body's carefully designed physiologic release of insulin. Therefore, though aggressive treatment of diabetes will lower the increased risk of cardiovascular disease and other effects, ultimately, the risk is still increased versus someone who is not diabetic. Therefore, the most successful treatment for diabetes is prevention or being able to eliminate the disease through lifestyle modification, which may be possible for type 2 diabetics.

Though the elimination of high blood pressure, high cholesterol, and diabetes is possible through appropriate diet and exercise for type 2 diabetics, the blood pressure and blood sugar issues make exercise more challenging. Those with high blood pressure who take blood pressure medicines may not be able to get as much blood flow to exercising muscles and tissues. Diabetics who take blood sugar-lowering medication may not have enough blood sugar to fuel the same tissues. These are just further reasons that prevention is the key, as medications can cause further issues that hinder your ability to implement all the lifestyle modifications necessary.

Other Effects

In addition to directly increasing your risk of cardiovascular disease, diabetes has many other devastating long-term effects on the body, some of which further increase your risk of suffering from cardiovascular disease.

In terms of some of diabetes' direct effects, the elevated blood sugar is known to cause neuropathy or disease of the nerves. In your legs, this can cause decreased sensation. Such decreased sensation can keep you from noticing and tending to minor injuries of your feet. Combine this with diabetics' poor ability to heal, and they are much more prone to infection. The neuropathy also tends to go into the optic nerve, which is responsible for our ability to see. For this reason, diabetics tend to have many more issues with vision.

Like high blood pressure, diabetes also affects the kidneys, and since the kidneys regulate blood pressure, this can contribute to high blood pressure. Once again, we see how certain risk factors for cardiovascular disease can worsen other risk factors. This is partly why people with multiple risk factors are at far greater risk than the total of the risks from each risk factor.

Get to Know Your Blood Sugar

You can determine whether you have diabetes by having the levels of glucose in the bloodstream measured. This is one of the simplest and most common tests for health care workers to perform, even simpler than cholesterol.

The Test

Though blood can be drawn to check for diabetes, similar to most other blood tests, a check for diabetes can actually be done with just a drop of blood from a simple prick of the finger and takes at most several minutes. The test is so common and easy that diabetics perform it themselves all the time to estimate how much insulin they need to give.

A normal result for a fasting glucose test is 65–109 mg/dL. A result that is 110–125 mg/dL could indicate an impaired fasting glucose level, also known as prediabetes. Like prehypertension, this may require more frequent monitoring or lifestyle changes. A result that is higher than 126 mg/dL could indicate diabetes.

ALERT

Prediabetes, or impaired fasting glucose, is a condition characterized by higher-than-normal blood glucose levels that are not high enough for diagnosis as type 2 diabetes. The American Diabetes Association (ADA) estimates that almost 20 million Americans have prediabetes. If you have this condition, work with your physician right away to start taking steps to lower your blood sugar levels.

Another way to test your blood glucose levels is with a hemoglobin A1C test. Unlike the finger-prick test, which provides a measure of your blood sugar at the moment of the test, the hemoglobin A1C shows your blood sugar levels over the past three months by analyzing the hemoglobin—the protein molecule in red blood cells that carries oxygen from the lungs to the body's tissues and returns carbon dioxide to the lungs from the tissues—rather than just the sugar levels. In order to establish a diagnosis of diabetes, a hemoglobin A1C test is necessary. The hemoglobin A1C test requires a blood draw, and the results are not immediate.

FACT

Approximately 1 million people are diagnosed with diabetes every year. The percentage of American adults with diagnosed diabetes, including women with a history of gestational diabetes (diabetes during pregnancy), has soared over the past two decades. Minority racial and ethnic populations are particularly at risk of developing the disease.

The American Diabetes Association recommends that people with diabetes take the hemoglobin A1C test two to four times a year. The test does not replace daily self-testing; rather, it provides a method to assess your success with blood sugar management over time. The U.S. Food and Drug Administration has approved a home test; check with your health care provider to see if it is appropriate for you.

Low Blood Sugar

Though having high blood sugar usually will not hurt you significantly over the short term but can be quite devastating over the long term, low blood sugar or hypoglycemia can be deadly in the short term. Like blood pressure, you need an adequate amount of blood sugar to sustain your body. Similar to low blood pressure, if your blood sugar gets too low you can suffer organ damage and death.

While blood pressure can get low for the variety of reasons mentioned previously, a person's blood sugar typically can't get so low on its own that it causes serious harm to the body. The only way for blood sugar to get so critically low is due to medications people take that artificially lower blood sugar. In other words, it's only diabetics that are at risk for low blood sugar.

Once again, this shows that addressing risk factors is important for multiple reasons. First, in addition to increasing your risk for cardiovascular disease, risk factors like diabetes have many other negative effects on the duration and quality of your life. Also, lifestyle modification is always the first choice for type 2 diabetics, as medications, despite being potentially helpful when used at the right time in the right way, can have many side effects, including deadly ones like low blood sugar. Finally, medications for diabetes will only address the risk of cardiovascular disease posed by blood sugar, while lifestyle modification can benefit your blood pressure, cholesterol, and blood sugar all at the same time, while having many other positive effects.

CHAPTER 5

Smoking

Smoking cigarettes greatly increases your risk of having a heart attack or stroke. Chemicals such as nicotine in cigarettes damage the lining of blood vessels and worsen your cholesterol. The good news is that within minutes of your last cigarette, your body starts to change for the better.

The Truth

You've probably already heard that smoking is bad for you. But do you really know what it can do? Consider the following facts: Smokers have a tremendously higher risk of lung diseases such as cancer, emphysema, bronchitis, and pulmonary fibrosis. Ever see people who have to walk around strolling an oxygen tank so they can breathe? Nearly all of those people became that way due to smoking. Imagine becoming out of breath after going only a few steps. Performing other tasks that help your life, like exercise, become tremendously harder.

The Many Effects of Smoking

Smoking also gives you a higher risk of nearly every form of cancer. In a healthy body, many areas have cells that go through a cycle of reproduction, where older cells die and newer cells take over. In cancer, some of the new cells have a genetic error where they end up replicating too much or living too long. The body makes more and more cells, ultimately creating a mass that can spread to invade your brain, lungs, liver, and bones.

FACT

Smoking is the cause of more than 440,000 deaths per year, according to the American Heart Association. This number represents more than one out of every six deaths!

Hurts You on Its Own

When compared with nonsmokers, smokers have twice the risk of having a heart attack or stroke, and even higher risk when other risk factors are present. Furthermore, smokers who have a heart attack are much more likely to die. Smoking increases the risk of sudden cardiac death.

How Smoking Hurts Your Heart

The mechanisms that cause cardiovascular disease from smoking and its many other devastating effects are still being researched, and it's for this reason that tobacco companies still often state there is no *direct* evidence showing how smoking causes so many diseases. Over the last several decades a huge amount of evidence emerged that linked smoking to many diseases, so much that even tobacco companies have begun to yield to all the research and admit that smoking causes health risks.

FACT

Smoking cigarettes is not only harmful to your lungs, it is also very damaging to the health of your heart and circulatory system. In fact, more smokers die from heart attacks and strokes than from lung cancer or respiratory disease.

It's widely believed that when inhaled, the many harmful substances in cigarettes get into the bloodstream and cause damage to arterial walls. As we have seen with high blood pressure, high cholesterol, and diabetes, this damage then fosters the formation of atherosclerosis and plaque formation, which then leads to issues such as heart attacks and strokes. Since all of these risk factors cause damage to blood vessel walls, it is easy to see how having several risk factors significantly raises your risk of cardiovascular disease.

Also, smokers tend to have a lower concentration of oxygen in their blood. Therefore, organs such as the heart do not receive the same amount of oxygen they would from blood flow. This decreased oxygen in the tissues hurts organ function, healing, and many other important processes. When the heart needs extra oxygen, as is often the case for people who develop cardiovascular disease, there is less oxygen to be supplied, contributing to the devastation from heart attacks and strokes.

ALERT

A recent surgeon general report states that the cellular damage and inflammation from smoking starts with the first cigarette, meaning there is no "safe" amount of smoking.

Smoking also increases inflammation of the lungs, causing or worsening diseases like asthma and emphysema, which cause difficulty breathing, lower oxygen in the lungs, and if untreated, death.

It Makes Everything Else Worse

Smoking does not just increase your risk of cardiovascular disease and work with other risk factors to further increase your risk, it can actually directly worsen your cholesterol and blood pressure as well.

Direct Effects

Cigarette smoking specifically harms the heart and circulatory system in a number of ways, including:

- Damaging the lining of the arteries
- Escalating heart rate and blood pressure by narrowing of the arteries
- Reducing the amount of available oxygen in the bloodstream by increasing levels of carbon monoxide, which compete with oxygen (and win) to bind with blood cells
- Raising the likelihood of blood-clot formation

So not only does smoking contribute to atherosclerosis and worsen some risk factors, it also increases the chance of forming a blood clot, which can clog blood vessels and contribute to a heart attack or stroke.

Indirect Effects

Blood vessels get stiffer when exposed to the toxins in cigarette smoke. Because of their stiffness, blood pressure increases. Also, blood vessels cannot dilate when necessary to meet increased oxygen and nutrient demands of organs, limiting blood flow to essential areas. This progressive formation of plaque that causes blood vessel thinning is a precursor to atherosclerosis.

In women, smoking increases the risk of ischemic strokes, intracerebral and subarachnoid hemorrhage, and problems with dangerous blood clots and burst blood vessels, according to the American Heart Association.

Not only does smoking decrease your HDL, it worsens the effect of LDL. In other words, cigarettes worsen your cholesterol profile in multiple ways.

Nonsmokers exposed to environmental tobacco smoke are at a 25 percent higher relative risk of developing heart disease than nonsmokers not exposed to environmental tobacco smoke. According to the American Heart Association, approximately 40,000 nonsmokers die each year from cardiovascular disease resulting from exposure to passive tobacco smoke. While you may find it impossible to completely prevent exposure to secondhand smoke, you will benefit from avoiding it as much as you can.

The Benefits of Quitting

By quitting smoking, you reduce your risk of heart disease. At the same time, your odds of developing disease will continue to decrease over the years. The benefits of quitting include less risk for numerous diseases including cardiovascular, and increased self-esteem and feelings of well-being. Quitting also benefits those around you who may suffer from consequences of secondhand smoke. Even if you believe that smoking in isolation cannot harm others, you track in many of the toxins on your body and clothing, which can still spread. If you smoke outside, you are spreading those toxins into the air that everyone breathes. If quitting for yourself is not enough, do it for others.

Quitting Improves Your Health

The health benefits of kicking the smoking habit truly start right away. Within twenty minutes of your last cigarette, nicotine is no longer causing constriction of blood vessels. As a result, your blood pressure decreases, your heart rate slows, and the temperature of your hands and feet rises as circulation improves. Within eight hours of your last cigarette, carbon monoxide levels drop in the bloodstream, and oxygen levels increase. Within twenty-four hours, the chances of having a heart attack are reduced. Within forty-eight hours, nerve endings begin to regenerate, and your sense of smell and taste start to return.

During the first year of not smoking, your body continues to heal itself from the stress of absorbing the cigarette toxins. Coughing, sinus congestion, fatigue, and shortness of breath start to fade as the strength of the lungs is restored. After a smoke-free year, the increased risk from smoking is cut in half. With each passing year, the risk continues to diminish.

Quitting the cigarette habit can improve your sex life. According to evidence from research, men who smoke fewer than ten cigarettes a day had a 16 percent higher risk of erectile dysfunction in comparison with men who had never smoked. Men who smoked more than one pack of cigarettes daily had a whopping 60 percent higher risk of erectile dysfunction when compared with nonsmokers.

Quitting Saves Time and Money

Another great benefit of quitting is that you will save quite a bit of money by giving up the cigarette habit. Your savings come mostly from the fact that you no longer need to buy cigarettes. Since smoking increases your risk for so many diseases, you also save money by staying healthy and not creating huge medical bills. In addition, you no longer need to spend time and effort looking for or buying cigarettes, lighters, and matches, or searching for places to light up.

It Does Not Just Help You

Not only will your improved health and energy help yourself, it will help those around you. Loved ones who smoke may become more inclined to quit, and by quitting you decrease the chance that nonsmokers will pick up the habit. By decreasing secondhand smoke exposure to those around you, you will improve their health as well. Their risk of cardiovascular disease and cancer will lower significantly. Sometimes it's challenging to do things for yourself, but when you quit smoking, you are also doing something great for others.

Getting Ready to Give Up Cigarettes

Approximately 70 percent of adult smokers want to quit. Quitting, however, is not easy. Many smokers try multiple times before they eventually succeed. Thorough preparation can increase your odds of achieving a smoke-free future. The federal government provides resources to assist people. In a program set forth on the website *www.smokefree.gov*, the preparatory phase consists of five steps represented by the acronym START.

The five steps are the following:

S = Set a quit date.
T = Tell family, friends, and coworkers that you plan to quit.
A = Anticipate and plan for the challenges that you will face.
R = Remove cigarettes and other tobacco products from your home, car, and work.
T = Talk to your doctor about getting help to quit.

The following sections examine each of these steps in detail.

Set a Quit Date

Once you have your mind made up that the benefits of not smoking far outweigh the risks of smoking, you are ready to set a quit date. Know that you are genuinely ready to make this commitment before you decide upon your quit date. Choose a specific day at least two weeks in advance. This gives you plenty of time to prepare, without losing your motivation to quit. Choose a day when you're best positioned to take that essential first step, such as when you are with others who can support you or at a place where you cannot get easy access to cigarettes.

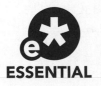
ESSENTIAL

If you smoke at work, it may make things easier on you if you select either a weekend or vacation day to get started. Or, to make the occasion more memorable, select a special occasion such as your birthday, anniversary, or a national holiday.

Tell Others Your Plan

Social support is the single most important factor in determining whether you are successful in changing poor habits into good ones. The help of your family and friends makes changing any behavioral pattern much easier.

Share your quitting plans with those who are close to you to solicit their support. It's often much harder to let others down than it is to let yourself down. Use peer pressure to your advantage.

The National Cancer Institute offers a smoking cessation guide with several helpful tips for developing your support system. First of all, the institute advises you to remind friends that your moods may change. Let them know that the longer you go without cigarettes, the sooner you will return to your old self. Also, if you have a friend or family member close to you who also smokes, see if he is interested in quitting with you. If not, ask him not to smoke around you. Seek out an ex-smoker to give you encouragement and advice during your tough moments.

Anticipate Challenges and Plan Ahead

Most people tend to form habitual patterns of smoking, such as immediately after a meal or when enjoying an alcoholic drink. These are the times that will present you with the strongest cravings. In addition to emotional cravings, most smokers also experience withdrawal symptoms including mood swings, feelings of irritability and depression, anxiety or restlessness, insomnia, headaches, difficulty concentrating, and increased hunger.

FACT

Consider joining a support group, either in person, on the phone, or in an Internet chat room. You can check with the American Cancer Society, the Heart Association, or Lung Association for leads on groups that you can join. Social support can provide a great way to help you quit.

These symptoms are worst the first few weeks, and they are extremely powerful during the first week of quitting. To help manage the cravings, use the time before you quit to concentrate on the moments you observe you want a cigarette most. Note when you have a cigarette and how you are feeling at the time. Then consider alternative ways to cope with those feelings and alternative activities during those times. For example, instead of having a cigarette after a meal, chew gum, drink water, squirt your mouth with breath spray, or brush your teeth. Be proactive in planning these alternatives, and buy the gum, breath spray, or whatever else you will need before you get to your scheduled quitting day.

If it is helpful to you to keep a journal, write down your observations. An even easier way to create this record of your smoking pattern is to wrap a piece of paper around your pack of cigarettes and secure it with a rubber band. Every time that you have a cigarette, write down the time of day, place, and your reason for having the cigarette. Later, take the list that you have created and write down alternative strategies for each of those instances. Once you recognize the situations where you are most likely to smoke, you can work to avoid or change those situations as much as possible.

Remove Cigarettes and Other Tobacco Products

Stop purchasing cartons of cigarettes. Don't save any packs as souvenirs of your willpower to quit. Those extra packs of cigarettes only make it all too easy to start smoking again.

Take a look around you. Take note of all the visual cues that support your smoking so you can start eliminating them from your environment. For example, throw out ashtrays, lighters, and matches. Remove the lighter in your car. Clean your home, office, and car by using air freshener and ridding all remnants of cigarette smoke. Make an appointment with your dentist to have your teeth cleaned and polished. Try to avoid close contact with those who are smoking or carry the smell of smoke.

Talk to Your Health Care Provider

Make sure you discuss your quitting plan with your health care provider. If you are taking any prescription medications, find out how changing your smoking habits may affect your medications.

Nicotine is powerfully addictive. There are medications that can help you avoid withdrawal symptoms. Enlist the support of your health care provider, and discuss your options together.

Aids to Stop Smoking

Many products exist today to aid the transition to a smoke-free life. Studies show that people who use nicotine replacement therapy are almost twice as successful as those who do not. Some smoking-cessation aids are available over the counter; others require a prescription.

ALERT

Consult with your health care provider before you start using any nicotine replacement therapy methods, as they can cause certain side effects. Pregnant women should be particularly cautious and work closely with their physician.

Nicotine Gum, Lozenges, and Patches

Nicotine gum, lozenges, and patches are available over the counter at your local pharmacy or grocery store. These products provide a low level of nicotine, without the accompanying toxins that come from smoking, to help you overcome the withdrawal symptoms.

The most common mistake people make with these products is not using enough. Do not skimp or underestimate the amount that you think you will need. Follow the directions on the package, and do not forget to continue to use your product. Over time, you can reduce the amount you use. Always keep some of the medication around to help you avoid cravings. Different medications work better for different people. The main advantage of gum is it provides oral stimulation, just as cigarettes do. Patches allow a slower form of release over a longer period of time.

Nicotine Inhalers and Nasal Sprays

Nicotine inhalers and nasal sprays both require a prescription from your doctor. Nasal sprays can provide immediate relief. Furthermore, sprays come in different concentrations, so you can reduce the amount of nicotine you put into your system over time.

Nicotine inhalers deliver nicotine into your system in much the same manner as cigarettes. For example, when you use a nicotine inhaler, you breathe the medication in through a mouthpiece. The nicotine is absorbed through the mouth's lining.

By using this inhalation technique, you most closely simulate the experience you had prior to smoking, allowing for an easier transition.

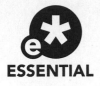
Bupropion

In contrast to the nicotine replacement therapies, bupropion pills, also known as Wellbutrin or Zyban, do not contain nicotine. Bupropion, originally developed as an antidepressant, was noticed to help reduce withdrawal symptoms and cigarette cravings. If you and your physician think this approach is good for you, you can even start taking the pill before your quit date.

This medication does require a prescription, however, and as it does have side effects, it is not appropriate for everyone. Medical experts recommend pregnant women, people with eating disorders, or people who experience seizures and drink heavily not use this medication.

Nicotine Poisoning

Take care not to smoke when you are using one of the nicotine replacement therapies. These products provide your body with nicotine, and it is possible to overdose. The signs of nicotine poisoning can include severe headaches, weakness, dizziness, nausea, vomiting, diarrhea, cold sweats, blurred vision, hearing difficulties, or mental confusion.

QUESTION

What should I do if I think I have nicotine poisoning?
Contact your health care provider or go to an emergency room if you experience any of the symptoms of nicotine poisoning when you are using a nicotine replacement product and you smoke. If you have any of these symptoms from wearing the patch, remove it immediately and wash your skin with water.

After You Quit—Avoiding Relapse

Quitting the cigarette habit is among the most challenging tasks that you will face. Be prepared, particularly in the first few days and weeks, to have alternate plans to keep you busy and to help you avoid dwelling on your urges to have a cigarette. Those times of day when you are accustomed to sitting back and lighting up will require special preparation. Here are some suggestions for other ways to use this time:

- Take a walk.
- Allow yourself time for a nap.
- Have some healthy snacks around to chew on.
- Drink lots of water.
- Chew gum or suck on candy.
- Use breath spray.
- Perform breathing exercises.
- Hold something in your hand, like a pencil.
- Pick up a craft like knitting or crocheting to keep your hands busy.
- Exercise to reproduce the neurotransmitter stimulation.
- Enjoy a hot bath.
- Listen to music.
- Spend time with or call supportive friends.
- Buy yourself some fun magazines or a good book that you want to read.
- Visit public places where smoking is not allowed so that you cannot light up.

Certain pastimes are also best avoided in these first few critical weeks. To help you stay away from these triggers:

- Keep away from drinking alcoholic beverages.
- Limit caffeinated beverages, as too many can make you feel tense.
- Pass up invitations to spend time with people who smoke.
- If you must spend time with smokers, immediately inform them that you have quit.
- Practice refusing the offer of a cigarette so you will have your reply prepared.

- Steer clear of places where other people are smoking.
- Eat regularly, and include snacks to avoid extreme feelings of hunger.
- Surround yourself with supportive friends and family, and stay away from circumstances that inflame strong emotions such as anger, resentment, or loneliness.
- Avoid high-stress situations as much as possible.
- Try not to push yourself into feeling overly tired.
- Pamper and spoil yourself, and indulge in other pleasures.

When a strong smoking urge strikes, immediately engage in one of your alternate activities. If you find yourself daydreaming about smoking, turn your thoughts to another subject. Continue to remind yourself of all the great benefits that you will experience once you have quit your habit. Exercise and meditate to increase positive feelings and reduce stress. Post visual reminders—photos of loved ones or whatever motivates you—to keep you on track with your goal.

If you do slip up, stop and forgive yourself. Get right back on your program. Remember that one cigarette is less harmful than an entire pack. Remind yourself that you can succeed and that you have strong reasons to quit smoking.

Smoke-Free for Life

Nicotine can be as addicting as heroin, so give yourself plenty of pats on the back for quitting and staying that way. It is quite an accomplishment, and you deserve a reward. One tangible way that you can reward yourself is to set aside a quit jar, where you put all the money you would normally have spent on your smoking habit. As often as you used to go out and buy a pack of cigarettes, put the money you would have used into your jar. After one month, take all the funds and indulge yourself by buying something purely for fun. Keep up this reward practice as long as you need that type of incentive and reminder not to start again.

Another critical factor is to follow the instructions of your nicotine replacement medication, if you are using one to assist you with quitting. A common mistake is for people to discontinue using the patch or gum a little sooner than recommended because they feel they have successfully overcome the urge to smoke. This can often lead to a relapse. Avoid this temptation. The first few months may remain challenging, so give yourself the extra support.

Another behavior that often leads to a relapse is the thought, "I'll just have one more. What can it hurt?" Studies show that even one more cigarette can often lead to a relapse and the need to repeat the difficult process of quitting. Remind yourself that the toughest time is those first few weeks, and that you do not want to go through the challenging process again. If it helps, write down the reasons you want to quit and post them in a visible place. Think about the health of yourself and others and the effects of your health on others.

FACT

Nicotine is a poison. If infants, children, or pets come into contact with or eat a nicotine patch, even a used one, it can cause serious harm. This is a medical emergency. If this occurs, contact your health care provider, emergency department, or poison control center immediately. Consider this another powerful reason to quit your habit as soon as possible.

Starting a new exercise program can often help you stay smoke-free. A walking program is not only easy, it can also improve your health and allow you to enjoy the feeling of taking deep breaths and the smell of fresh air. Regular walking can also help with managing any extra weight gain that resulted from kicking the smoking habit. Exercise releases many of the same stimulants and neurotransmitters of smoking, making the quitting process easier. It also helps reduce stress, further reducing the temptation to light up. Other methods of reducing stress, such as meditation and relaxation, can similarly help reduce those urges.

Simply take a moment to truly acknowledge the power of your own convictions to create better health for yourself. Take each day one step at a time. Congratulate yourself for choosing health, not only for yourself, but also for your loved ones and everyone else around you.

CHAPTER 6

Testing

The reason for getting tested is to understand your risk for developing heart disease, stroke, or any of the other consequences of atherosclerosis. Poor cholesterol, high blood pressure, or diabetes often have no visible symptoms. The only way to learn whether you are at higher risk for a heart attack or stroke is to get yourself tested. You can get tested in your medical doctor's office, at a medical laboratory, or at public screenings.

When to Get Checked

Although risk factors alone are not predictive of heart disease in all people, knowing your risk is a valuable first step. When you know your risks, you gain valuable insight into the health of your current lifestyle and what you need to do to become or stay healthy. Furthermore, for those people who learn that they fall into high-risk categories, the sooner they begin a treatment plan to lower levels of bad cholesterol and increase levels of good cholesterol, the sooner they can start to reduce their risks of heart attack or stroke.

Cholesterol Testing

Federal government guidelines recommend that all Americans check their cholesterol levels with a complete fasting lipoprotein profile at the age of twenty. The measurements taken by this test include your levels of total cholesterol, HDL cholesterol, LDL cholesterol, and triglycerides. If test results indicate that all levels are in a healthy range, then government guidelines recommend retesting at a minimum of every five years. The full lipoprotein profile test is preferred over a test that provides data regarding only total cholesterol and HDL levels, because knowing LDL cholesterol and triglycerides allows medical providers to better target adjustments in lifestyle and medical therapy. Regular blood pressure screenings, blood sugar checks, and physical exams are also recommended to better screen your overall health and cardiovascular risk.

If you do not fast at least nine to twelve hours before testing your cholesterol, you can measure only total cholesterol and HDL levels. To receive more detailed information regarding your levels of LDL cholesterol and triglycerides, fasting is necessary. The reason for fasting is that certain foods and alcohol will cause your cholesterol levels to spike.

Although federal government guidelines recommend cholesterol testing for adults at least every five years, if you have had a major change of lifestyle during that five-year period, your cholesterol levels may be different and, therefore, worth checking again before five full years elapse. For example, if you were a college student at age twenty and then became a working professional after graduation at age twenty-one or twenty-two, your physical activity levels, dietary choices, and stress levels may have changed significantly. All of these factors can impact your cholesterol levels. Therefore, it may be worth your time and effort to know your numbers as a measure of your health status in your new lifestyle. In general, you should err on the side of caution and get your levels checked more often. Cholesterol testing is relatively quick and inexpensive and reveals very valuable information.

Under current government guidelines, if you fall into a category that requires treatment for your cholesterol levels, you will have your cholesterol tested at much more frequent intervals to evaluate the success of the treatment program and to make any necessary adjustments. Subsequent visits for additional monitoring and adjustment of therapy should be scheduled at appropriate intervals depending on the nature of the individual therapy. Typically, if your cholesterol is in the borderline dangerous range, you should have a recheck in approximately six months. How often you receive subsequent rechecks will be based on your levels during the initial recheck and the opinion of your medical provider.

Blood Pressure Testing

For almost everyone, blood pressure is checked very often. It's checked in almost any health care setting, whether a clinic visit, in the emergency department, even often at the dentist or when donating blood. Because of this, people often know if their blood pressure runs high. If you have not had your blood pressure checked recently, use any of the free automatic blood pressure machines available at nearly every pharmacy. Though these automatic machines are slightly less accurate, and decisions regarding blood pressure should not be made just after one testing, getting this basic check can help gauge the urgency of getting follow-up. It's not just the test, it's what you do about it!

Blood Sugar Testing

As discussed, the test for blood sugar is perhaps the simplest of all blood tests, as it could be done with a simple prick of the finger. Despite this, there are many undiagnosed diabetics. The reason for this is because most people do not see their health care practitioner regularly enough. Unlike blood pressure, which is checked in many health care settings, your blood sugar is typically only checked in the setting of a physician visit.

ESSENTIAL

High blood pressure, high blood sugar, and a poor cholesterol profile are known as silent killers because often there are no symptoms. Because there are no symptoms, people often do not realize they have the disease and therefore do not seek treatment. Make sure you know your risk and get tested!

Another reason for less diagnosis is the guidelines for blood sugar testing are less official and publicized than cholesterol screening. Further, the lesser known guidelines do not recommend initial screening until the age of forty-five years old. Challenging these guidelines is outside the scope of this book, but if you do have concerns that you either have symptoms of diabetes or feel you are at higher risk due to lifestyle factors or a family history, do not hesitate to see a health care practitioner to perform the test. As mentioned, the test is simple and could save your life.

For known diabetics, an HbA1C level may be measured. This test measures how good your blood pressure control has been over the preceding three months by measuring how much sugar is stuck on the protein of your red blood cells, hemoglobin. As it's an average of several months, it's less prone to variability than simple blood sugar levels, and can be used to adjust diabetes medications.

Circumstances That Can Affect Your Test Results

Your general health also has an effect on your test results. Do not go ahead with a scheduled test if you have a cold or the flu. Cholesterol, blood sugar, and blood pressure can go up or down temporarily during periods of acute illness, immediately following a heart attack or stroke, or during acute stressors such as surgery or an accident. For a more accurate measure, medical experts recommend that you wait at least several weeks after an illness before getting checked.

Timing

The ideal time to obtain an accurate test is when you are observing your usual routine, as this would then accurately reflect your genetics and life-style. All of these test results may change daily in response to deviations from your normal physical activity and eating habits, particularly if you increase your fat intake. Rapid weight loss also impacts all of these tests. For the truest insight into your risk of heart disease, schedule your test at a time when you are living your typical, routine lifestyle.

ESSENTIAL

Current government guidelines suggest that the ideal LDL choles-terol level is 160 or lower if you have cardiovascular risk factors. In fact, for those with who are considered high-risk, ideal LDL levels are below 100.

The only exception to living your usual routine is fasting for at least nine hours prior to getting your blood sugar and cholesterol checked, so that the recent meal does not have too much of an influence on the levels. It's believed that the fasting blood sugar and blood cholesterol levels are bet-ter markers of your risk for heart disease. The best way to get a fasting test while living your typical routine is to get tested in the morning prior to your first meal of the day, as that's typically the longest time you go without food.

Influence of Prescription Drugs

Many medications may affect cholesterol levels. These medications include the following:

- ACTH (adrenocorticotropic hormone)
- Anabolic steroids
- Beta-adrenergic blocking agents (beta blockers)

- Corticosteroids
- Epinephrine
- Oral contraceptives
- Phenytoin
- Sulfonamides
- Thiazide diuretics
- Vitamin D

If you are taking any medications that have a potentially adverse impact on your cholesterol levels, be sure to discuss this with your health care provider. Make sure that you understand how you will monitor your cholesterol levels over time to ensure they remain within a healthy range.

Can You Know Too Much?

Most of this book is devoted to knowing information you may not have known previously. There is another extreme, though, and that is actually knowing your information too well. At a certain point, some negative effects of obsession with your health may outweigh the positive effects.

Variability

Many basic measures of health vary on a day-to-day basis. It is possible to check too frequently and react too hastily to results. Remember, an appropriate screening has you fasting for at least nine to twelve hours, and even when done appropriately, there remains some variability.

Your blood pressure, blood sugar, and cholesterol all vary every minute, hour, and day. Though practices like fasting while otherwise living your life with a similar routine decreases this variability and influence of recent behaviors, the variability exists nonetheless. This is why decisions are often not made based on an initial screening. For example, with blood pressure, it's well known that blood pressure readings tend to be higher in physician offices, especially on the first visit. This is so common it even has a name, white-coat hypertension, as it is likely due to the stress of the visit. Because of this phenomenon, physicians generally make sure to not make any decisions based on this first reading, and often repeat checks in either future visits or even check again during the first visit.

Stress

When you become overconsumed with measuring parameters of health, whether cholesterol, blood pressure, or blood sugar, you add to the body's stress levels, which may worsen all of these measures. As you know, stress is a risk factor for high blood pressure, high blood sugar, a poor cholesterol profile, and cardiovascular disease itself. Therefore, you do not want to act in any way that is going to add stress to your life.

While testing and being informed are important, far more important are your actions to improve your health, no matter what your test results are. These tests offer only some idea of the relative impact these essential actions will have. If you focus too much on the tests and lose sight of the goals of improving health and avoiding serious disease, then the testing becomes meaningless. Like any aspect of your health, the most important thing is finding the right balance.

Short-Term Versus Long-Term

Remember that, generally, high blood pressure, poor cholesterol, and diabetes are silent killers. This means that you do not typically feel the effects, and that the long-term damage is what's truly devastating. Despite this, when people have an abnormal test result, they tend to want to respond immediately. The key is remembering that poor test results will tend not to cause serious harm over a day, week, or month, but over years and years.

ESSENTIAL

Blood pressure, blood sugar, and cholesterol can vary due to many factors, or no factors at all. In order, this variability tends to be greatest in blood pressure, then blood sugar, then cholesterol. For all of these repeat testing is in order, though it's more important the greater the variability.

If you respond hastily to test results, you may do more harm than good. For example, when seeking a quick fix, you may ignore the far more beneficial lifestyle modification that can help improve all of your risk factors, and simply want to take a medication. The problem with this approach is that medication will only address the single risk factor. Furthermore, if decisions are made based on a single test result, not accounting for the constant changes in your body, there can be an overcorrection, which is far more dangerous than the abnormal test result. For example, while high blood pressure and high blood sugar are dangerous over the course of years, low blood pressure and low blood sugar can be deadly immediately.

Rather than trying to immediately overcompensate for any abnormal test results, consider results over time and in the right testing conditions. Let your experienced health care providers be your guide, as they understand all the risks and benefits and can ensure that any action taken is appropriate.

What Your Test Results Mean

Knowing is only half the battle; what matters even more is what you do with this information. Most of this section will be devoted to your cholesterol test results, because your cholesterol results represent your entire lipid profile rather than just one number, like your blood pressure and blood sugar.

Cholesterol Results

In general, the higher your total blood cholesterol level, the greater your risk of heart disease. For example, a person with a total cholesterol level of 240 mg/dL may have as much as twice the risk of heart disease as someone with a total cholesterol level of less than 200 mg/dL.

Total cholesterol alone does not tell the complete story. Heart disease risk is related to the composition of your total cholesterol. For example, if you have high total cholesterol due to a very high HDL level, then that is a positive condition. On the other hand, if your total cholesterol is not high, but you have a high LDL level or a low HDL level, then that is a negative condition. Unfortunately, for most people, having a high total cholesterol means they have a high LDL level; rarely will high total cholesterol be due to high

HDL. This is why high total cholesterol likely means you are at higher risk for heart disease.

ESSENTIAL

Research shows that high levels of total cholesterol are indicators of future heart problems. Total cholesterol, however, is composed mostly of LDL particles. Therefore, leading experts believe that the strong relationship between total cholesterol and heart disease is reflective of the fact that high LDL levels are a risk factor.

Those who have cholesterol levels 200–239 mg/dL are considered to have borderline high risk. However, this is not necessarily cause for alarm. If total cholesterol levels are high because of high HDL levels of more than 60 mg/dL, it actually means that you have a reduced risk of heart disease, assuming that you have no other risk factors.

People with total cholesterol levels of 240 mg/dL are classified as high risk, as levels this elevated are almost always due to LDL.

LDL Cholesterol

High levels of LDL cholesterol are known to be a major cause of heart disease. Federal government guidelines focus on reducing LDL levels as the primary means of providing therapy for people with high cholesterol. Strong research evidence supports the idea that reducing LDL levels results in reducing the risk of heart disease. The following table reflects the classification of LDL cholesterol levels that are recommended by both the federal government and the American Heart Association for adults.

▼ **CLASSIFICATION OF LDL CHOLESTEROL LEVELS FOR ADULTS**

LDL Cholesterol		Category
Less than 100 mg/dL	2.5	Optimal
100–129 mg/dL	3.2	Near optimal
130–159 mg/dL	4.0	Borderline
160–189 mg/dL	4.7	High
Above 189 mg/dL	4.7	Very high

Current treatment approaches for people with high total cholesterol levels are based on LDL levels, other risk factors, and the calculated percentage of short-term risk of having heart disease. People with elevated cholesterol levels are classified into three categories of risk for treatment.

An existing diagnosis of coronary artery disease or an equivalent condition is a very important factor that affects the treatment goal for LDL-lowering therapy. If the following conditions are present, the individual is considered to fall into the highest category of risk and is therefore recommended to receive the most aggressive therapeutic treatment to achieve an LDL of less than 100mg/dL or lower:

- Known coronary artery disease
- Other forms of cardiovascular disease, such as peripheral arterial disease, abdominal aortic aneurysm, and symptomatic carotid artery disease
- Diabetes
- Two or more other risk factors

These other risk factors include:

- Smoking
- Age: males over forty-five years old or females over fifty-five years old
- HDL less than 40 mg/dL
- Having a first-degree relative with premature heart disease (males over fifty-five years old, females over sixty-five years old)
- Hypertension

If you have only one of the Framingham risk factors without coronary artery disease or one of its equivalents, you are in the moderate-risk category and your recommended LDL is less than 130 mg/dL. If you have none, then you are considered low risk and want to maintain an LDL level below 160 mg/dL, the cutoff for high cholesterol.

To summarize, if you are without any risk factors, you are considered low risk and your LDL goal is 160 mg/dL. If you have one of the risk factors of age, you are at moderate risk and your LDL goal is 130 mg/dL. If you have two of these risk factors or if you have diabetes, coronary artery disease, or its equivalent, you are high risk and your LDL goal is 100 mg/dL or lower.

These recommendations are not absolute. New, slightly adjusted recommendations are constantly being proposed and fine-tuned. Your health care provider may further subclassify you and your risk and individually tailor your treatment goals and therapy. These guidelines are meant to give you a general idea of your cardiovascular risk and cholesterol goals.

HDL Cholesterol

Levels of HDL or good cholesterol show an inverse relationship to heart disease risk. Remember, HDL cholesterol acts as the transporter that takes cholesterol away from the blood vessels and back to the liver for metabolizing. Unlike LDL cholesterol and triglycerides, where high numbers mean increased risk, higher levels of HDL cholesterol mean a lower risk of heart disease. There are more transporters taking cholesterol away from the arteries, leading to less plaque buildup and clogging. In healthy individuals, HDL cholesterol represents approximately 20–30 percent of total cholesterol levels. Since HDL is only a minor fraction and has a narrower range, elevated total cholesterol is typically due to elevated LDL and is considered a risk factor for cardiovascular disease.

Researchers have found that some individuals whose lower levels of HDL are due to genetic disorders also have a higher risk of heart disease. Again, genes can influence risk of heart disease, and they show why family history is important in determining your own risk.

Some scientists believe there may be multiple subtypes of HDL cholesterol, just as there are multiple subtypes of LDL cholesterol, and that some subtypes of HDL have more beneficial characteristics than others. In general, elevated HDL is a negative risk factor, but HDL levels that are too low are a risk to your health.

Evidence from studies shows that low HDL cholesterol is an independent risk factor for heart disease. This means that regardless of whether other risk factors are present, the risk of heart disease is higher for people with low HDL. This is why HDL is a listed risk factor in determining the need for LDL therapy. A 1 percent decrease in HDL levels is associated with a 2–3 percent increase in heart disease risk. The following chart sets forth the classification of HDL cholesterol levels as adopted by federal government guidelines and the American Heart Association:

▼ **CLASSIFICATION OF HDL CHOLESTEROL LEVELS FOR ADULTS**

HDL Cholesterol Levels	Classification	Risk Category
Less than 40 mg/dL <1	Low HDL cholesterol	High risk
40–59 mg/dL 1.5	Moderate HDL cholesterol	Higher levels are desirable
60 mg/dL and above >1.5	High LDL cholesterol	Negative risk factor

Interestingly, adult women tend to have higher HDL levels than adult men, likely due to hormonal influences. According to government estimates, approximately one-third of all adult men and one-fifth of adult women have low HDL levels that put them at increased risk of heart disease. At 40 mg/dL, however, both men and women are considered to have low HDL—there is no separate recommendation for women. Nor is there a separate recommendation regarding HDL levels for children.

Natural strategies to increase HDL include losing weight, increasing activity, and quitting smoking. Of these, exercise seems to have the most significant effect on HDL. These natural strategies have positive effects, including boosting energy and increasing strength, as opposed to the harmful side effects created by some prescription drugs.

ESSENTIAL

Some medications that lower LDL cholesterol also raise HDL levels, giving twice the bang for the buck. Medications, of course, come with their own risks, so be sure to discuss these risks with your doctor.

The term negative risk factor refers to the fact that high HDL cholesterol is such a positive condition that it actually "negates" one of the other risk factors. For example, elevated HDL cholesterol might cancel out the risk from having elevated blood pressure. Despite "canceling" the risk, you can reduce your risk the most by having elevated HDL with no other risk factors.

Triglyceride Results

Triglycerides are a form of fat. Their structure is made up of three fatty acids attached to glycerol. Triglycerides are present in most fatty foods and are the most common fat in the body. Triglycerides that float in the bloodstream provide fuel for energy when your sugar stores run low. Those that are not used for fuel are stored in the body's fatty tissues. Recent research has made it clear that high triglyceride levels are a marker for increased risk of heart disease and are possibly an independent risk factor. In addition, high triglycerides are usually present when other risk factors, such as diabetes and high LDL cholesterol, are present. Triglycerides make up a main component of VLDL, or very low-density lipoprotein. Like LDL, these low-density lipoproteins can form atherosclerosis and plaques and cause the same health risks.

As the role of triglycerides in the process of developing heart disease becomes clearer, experts support efforts to keep triglyceride levels low. The federal government and the American Heart Association have come up with the following guidelines regarding fasting blood levels of triglycerides in adults:

▼ CLASSIFICATIONS OF TRIGLYCERIDE LEVELS

Triglyceride Level	Classification
Less than 150 mg/dL	Normal
150–199 mg/dL	Borderline high
200–499 mg/dL	High
Above 499 mg/dL	Very high

As with low HDL and high LDL levels, behavioral factors are the root cause of high triglyceride levels. Excess weight and lack of physical activity are the most common causes. However, any of the following can be a factor: cigarette smoking; excess alcohol consumption; very high carbohydrate intake levels (more than 60 percent of total calories per day); drugs such as beta-blockers, corticosteroids, estrogens, and protease inhibitors for HIV; heredity; or other diseases such as type 2 diabetes, chronic renal failure, and nephrotic syndrome. Notice that many contributors on this list are the same contributors to poor HDL and LDL levels, as well as independent risk factors for cardiovascular disease itself. People who do not have any of these factors generally have triglyceride levels of less than 100 mg/dL. As with LDL and HDL, the first course of action to lower triglyceride levels is to adopt lifestyle changes, including improved nutrition and increased physical activity.

Total Cholesterol and HDL Ratio

Since total cholesterol is primarily composed of HDL and LDL, for a quick estimation of risk, you can calculate your total cholesterol and HDL ratio. To do this, divide your total cholesterol number by your HDL number. This method is based on the fact that high HDL levels relative to your total cholesterol are generally predictive of a lower risk of heart disease. While this estimate can give you a rough idea of your cholesterol-level breakdown, it is not recommended as a test upon which to base therapeutic treatment.

Today, the American Heart Association uses absolute numbers for LDL and HDL cholesterol levels. They are more useful to physicians than the cholesterol ratio in determining appropriate treatment for patients. If you're interested in calculating your ratio, the classifications are as follows:

▼ **CLASSIFICATIONS OF RATIO OF TOTAL CHOLESTEROL TO HDL**

TC/HDL Ratio	Classification
3.5 to 1	Optimum
4.5 to 1	Desirable
5 to 1 and above	High

To apply the formula, let's take an example of a woman with a total cholesterol level of 200 and an HDL level of 50. Her ratio is calculated by dividing 200 by 50, to equal a ratio of 4 to 1. According to this rough measure, her cholesterol is in the desirable range, but for a more comprehensive understanding, it's necessary to look at the entire spectrum of blood lipid levels.

Blood Pressure Results

Blood pressure is much simpler to interpret than cholesterol because it's only two numbers. The upper number, or systolic blood pressure, is the pressure with which the heart pumps and blood exerts on blood vessels when the heart is contracting. The lower number, or diastolic blood pressure, is the pressure exerted when the heart is relaxed.

High blood pressure is defined as a blood pressure reading over 140/90 mmHg. If just one of the two numbers is above this, you are considered to have high blood pressure.

Over years, blood pressures creep steadily higher for the many reasons discussed, especially the hardening of our blood vessels. This makes high blood pressure one of the most prevalent diseases in society, and because of the long-term impact it can have, one of the deadliest. Because of this and the fact the blood pressure can be so easily tested, it's the risk factor that people know about best and tend to respond to the most.

If a blood pressure measurement is taken and either the systolic or diastolic blood pressure is elevated, it's important that repeat measurements be taken by a health care provider. If the blood pressure is persistently elevated, as with all risk factors, the first step is lifestyle modification through diet, exercise, and stress reduction. If blood pressure remains elevated on repeat measurements by health care providers despite such lifestyle changes, then medications should be considered.

Recently, more attention has been paid to the prehypertensive zone, or a blood pressure above 120/80mmHg. Though this is under the cut-off for a diagnosis of hypertension, it is felt there may be some benefit from lowering blood pressure below this value in higher-risk people or people who have other risk factors. In other words, if you are higher risk for heart disease with multiple risk factors, similar recommendations apply to those with a diagnosis of hypertension. Lifestyle modification comes first, but then medication may be considered.

Blood Sugar Results

Though testing for blood sugar is not quite as simple and readily available as blood pressure testing, as blood pressure testing is noninvasive, blood sugar remains the simplest blood test there is. It can be performed with a prick of the finger and the results are immediate. Its simplicity is reflected in the number and frequency that people check their own blood sugars at home. You should not check your own blood sugar outside of the health care setting for a diagnosis unless a health care provider specifically instructs you to do so.

If your fasting blood sugar is above 126 mg/dL on repeat measurements by a health care provider, then you will likely be diagnosed with diabetes. Like with blood pressure, this means you should begin lifestyle modification consisting of diet, exercise, and stress reduction. In the case of diabetes, dietary modification becomes the most important. Read future chapters for discussions on how to improve one's diet as well other types of lifestyle modification.

Similar to a prehypertensive zone, there is a zone of prediabetes consisting of a fasting blood sugar 100–125 mg/dL. Having a fasting blood sugar in the prediabetes zone is highly predictive of being diagnosed with type 2 diabetes within the next ten years, requiring a similar urgency in intervening with lifestyle modification and, if necessary, medication.

FACT

There are actually several different types of blood sugar tests for diabetes, though the most commonly used is the fasting blood sugar, as it has a balance of accuracy and simplicity. In rare cases, your healthcare provider may choose to use one of the alternative tests.

Fasting blood sugars tend to be far more accurate than random blood sugars, but a random blood sugar above 200 mg/dL suggests the diagnosis of diabetes. There exists a more complicated but slightly more accurate oral glucose tolerance test, where a blood sugar is drawn two hours after ingestion of a 75g sugar solution. Below 139 mg/dL is considered normal, 140–199 mg/dL is prediabetic, and over 200 mg/dL is diabetes.

Other Tests for Your Heart

Your health care provider may include some of these tests as part of a routine physical checkup. In addition to these tests, medical professionals may use other tests to achieve a full picture of the health of the heart and circulatory system.

Noninvasive Diagnostic Tests

Several of the tests doctors use to measure the function of the heart and the state of the arteries are noninvasive, meaning they are done without entering the body or puncturing the skin. Instead, medical professionals use different types of technology to look at the heart and arteries and to measure how well they are functioning. These tests are typically performed on those considered at higher risk for cardiovascular disease.

In the stress test, you exercise on a treadmill or a stationary bicycle to put your heart under stress. As you are exercising, medical professionals will administer tests to measure your heart's response to the stress and ensure your arteries are not so clogged that you do not have adequate blood flow to meet the demand. An electrocardiogram (EKG), which measures the electrical flow through your heart, monitors your heart during the test. The test involves putting electrodes on your chest that are connected to a machine, the electrocardiograph. The electrocardiograph prints out a record of how the heart is beating and reveals any irregularities. As you exercise, the printout shows whether your heart is able to meet the extra demand placed on it by the exercise.

ALERT

Studies show that some diagnostic tests and procedures are not as accurate in women as in men. For example, an exercise stress test may show a false positive or negative, but this is more likely in a younger woman. Some doctors prefer other types of tests that are more diagnostically accurate for young women.

Due to certain physical conditions, some individuals cannot undergo the rigors of a stress test. In these cases, doctors use medications to stress the heart as if it were exercising. They then follow the flow of the tracer and assess the health of the heart and its coronary arteries.

An echocardiogram, also known as an "echo" test or EKG, uses sound waves to take a dynamic picture of the heart as it beats. An ultrasound transducer transmits high-frequency sound waves directed toward the heart. The cardiologist analyzes this moving picture of the heart to evaluate its functioning. Echocardiography reveals the shape and thickness of the walls in the heart's chambers and the large veins and arteries of the heart, among other things. Medical professionals also use echocardiography with stress tests, performing the echo before the stress test begins and immediately after it stops.

Magnetic resonance imaging (MRI) and computed tomography (CT) are other noninvasive tests. These tests use a magnet and/or radiofrequency waves to read signals from the body's cells to create an image of the interior of the body. To take the test, the patient lies on a mobile examination table that moves through a large tube. The cardiologist analyzes the MRI images and data to evaluate the blood supply to the heart muscle and to assess the function of the blood vessels. In certain CT scans, the image reader can see calcium from plaques within the arteries that feed the heart muscle blood and oxygen.

ESSENTIAL

The tests described can provide you with some insight into the true state of plaque buildup within your arteries. This information can help you refine the degree of risk for an imminent heart attack, but none of the tests is perfect or takes away the risk of cardiovascular disease. No matter what the results show, risk-factor modification remains key.

Invasive Testing

An angiogram is an invasive test used to measure the degree of blockage in blood vessels. It is considered the best way to detect narrowing of blood vessels, but due to the risk of the procedure, it is done only in very high-risk individuals. To perform an angiogram, the physician punctures a major artery and inserts a long plastic catheter up to a heart blood vessel. Then a dye is injected into the catheter to allow for observation of the heart blood vessels. The doctor observes the dye's progress on an X-ray machine to see how it flows through the vessels.

If the angiogram reveals a blockage, the doctor may perform an angioplasty, which involves clearing the blockage from the artery and then placing a hollow tube, called a stent, on the inside of the blood vessel to keep it open. If the blockage is so severe that the artery cannot be saved, surgery to create a bypass to the blocked vessel may be required.

Intravascular ultrasound (IVUS) uses sound waves to create a multi-dimensional image that shows the level of blood flow and plaque buildup inside the coronary artery. Medical professionals take images using a catheter with a transducer inside the artery itself. This can provide an extremely accurate view of the size of the vessel's opening and condition of the plaque and arterial walls, but this technology is still in the early stages of development.

Another method of stress testing uses a radioactive tracer that is injected intravenously. The tracer flows through the arteries. Medical professionals use special cameras to view the tracer's passage as it reveals the extent of openness or blockage of various blood vessels.

Blood Tests

The presence of higher-than-normal levels of C-reactive protein (CRP) or highly specific CRP (hsCRP) in the bloodstream is nonspecific evidence of an infectious or inflammatory disease in the body. CRP is not indicative of the presence of a specific disease but simply that the body is fighting some form of infection or inflammation.

Strong evidence from research studies shows that CRP is also a marker for heart disease. Women with high CRP levels were five times more likely than women with low CRP levels to develop heart disease and seven times more likely to have a stroke or heart attack. Again, an elevated CRP does not give any specific information, nor does a normal CRP rule out disease. CRP may only raise or lower the chance that a disease is occurring.

The reason that CRP levels can be a marker for heart disease is related to the fact that damage to or inflammation of the interior lining of the arteries (referred to as the endothelial lining) precedes the formation of plaque. In other words, plaque collects in locations where there is damage to arterial walls. CRP can be evidence of this damage.

When LDL cholesterol combines with a substance known as apolipoprotein (a), the result is a compound known as Lp(a), which can increase your risk of heart attack or stroke. Federal government guidelines describe Lp(a) as an emerging risk factor. Researchers believe that the presence of Lp(a) can increase the formation of blood clots and the formation of plaque by assisting LDL particles attach to plaque buildups.

ESSENTIAL

Approximately 50 percent of people who have heart attacks do not have elevated cholesterol levels. These individuals, however, typically have higher levels of CRP, Lp(a), or other potential markers such as apo B or homocysteine. As researchers continue to learn about the exact mechanisms of heart disease, more tests are developed to identify and measure these other risk factors and markers.

Genetics determines your levels of Lp(a) and even the size of the Lp(a) molecule itself. Lifestyle changes do not alter levels of Lp(a); instead, levels for most people tend to remain consistent over a lifetime, except for women, who will experience a slight rise in levels with menopause. Some physicians request testing of Lp(a) for patients who have a strong family history of premature heart disease.

Treatment for elevated Lp(a) includes niacin therapy and concentrating efforts on lowering LDL levels, because at lower levels, it is harder for LDL particles to attach to plaque buildup.

CHAPTER 7

Drug Therapy

Reducing your risk of cardiovascular disease, disability, and death requires that you make a commitment to support and enhance healthful living. Medications support this process. Drugs can be valuable tools to help you achieve optimal health. For some people, drug therapy to manage lipid levels is the best short-term action, until lifestyle changes have time to improve cardiovascular health. For others, drug therapy is the only way to address genetic tendencies toward unhealthy lipid levels.

When to Use Drugs

As you read about side effects, keep in mind that pharmaceuticals are potentially very beneficial. Do not become alarmed by precautions and necessary safeguards—it's important to have information to make intelligent choices. Medications, like most medical interventions, require an examination of the risk versus benefit. This is why medications are often considered only after lifestyle changes.

Studies show that drug therapy is more effective when used together with lifestyle changes to achieve healthy cholesterol levels and reduce the risk of heart attack and stroke. When you incorporate a multipronged approach, you get results more quickly, you are able to reduce your medication levels sooner, and you will feel the improvements in your health more rapidly.

ESSENTIAL

Though medications may be an important part of risk-factor modification, lifestyle modification always comes first. Not only will adjusting your lifestyle benefit multiple risk factors, but unlike medications, the side effects are only positive ones.

Your physician may prescribe combination drug therapy, depending on the risk factors and whether you already have heart disease. The target cholesterol, blood pressure, or blood sugar is more aggressive for people with certain existing problems. To achieve this low level, your physician may prescribe a combination of medications in addition to lifestyle changes. Depending on the combination of drugs, side effects may decrease due to needing a lower dosage of each drug or increase due to drug interactions.

When you are put on therapeutic medications, your physician will regularly monitor your blood pressure, blood sugar, or cholesterol levels to ascertain your progress. If you do not reach your goal after three months with a single drug, your doctor may recommend a second medicine to improve your progress. If you report particular side effects to your physician, she may also prescribe lower doses of a combination of medications to lessen the possibility of adverse effects.

Should You Take an Aspirin a Day?

As most heart attacks and strokes are caused by blood clots, more attention has been given to medications that help prevent blood clots to possibly prevent these devastating diseases. Blood thinners, such as Heparin and Coumadin, have not been shown to significantly reduce the chances of having a heart attack or stroke. Antiplatelet drugs, the most well known being aspirin, have been shown to have such an effect. There are other antiplatelet medications as well, but these are only available by prescription and generally for certain people who are extremely high risk, such as those who have had heart attacks and/or have an aspirin allergy.

Because aspirin is over the counter, many people choose to self-medicate because they believe it will prevent certain cardiovascular diseases. Doing this may not be the best idea, though. First of all, aspirin has not been shown to significantly affect the process of atherosclerosis, the main precursor to vessel blockages. Also, aspirin, despite being over the counter, has many side effects. Aspirin can cause gastrointestinal bleeding as well as increase bleeding everywhere else in the body, due to its anticlotting effects. These risks can outweigh the benefits in those who are not at least moderate risk for heart disease. In addition, most people are not sure how much aspirin they should take. Discuss with your doctor whether you believe you should take an aspirin, and if so, the recommended dosage.

Cholesterol Drugs

This section provides an overview of the various drugs frequently prescribed to manage lipids, such as statins, bile acid sequestrants, nicotinic acid, and fibrates. These are the most common drugs prescribed to treat cholesterol, either alone or in combination.

Statins, Your First Line of Defense

Statins are usually the drugs of choice for improving cholesterol levels. The primary goal of all lipid therapy is reduction of LDL cholesterol. Since statins lower LDL more than any other type of drug, while raising HDL and lowering triglycerdies, physicians typically consider them first. Statins, like many lifestyle changes, improve all aspects of your lipid profile and therefore have the most beneficial cardiovascular effect. Statins are typically the least prone to side effects of various medical therapies, despite still having significant potential effects.

Statins accomplish this reduction of LDL by blocking an enzyme, HMG-CoA reductase, which produces cholesterol in the liver. With this enzyme inhibited, the liver manufactures less cholesterol. Since the liver needs cholesterol, it removes more cholesterol from the bloodstream to replace what it is blocked from making. In this manner, statins reduce LDL production and also boost the body's ability to remove excess LDL circulating in the bloodstream.

Depending on the dosage, statins have shown the ability to greatly reduce LDL levels; aggressive statin therapy has proved to reduce cardiac risk in very high-risk individuals by up to 60 percent and stroke risk by almost 20 percent. A higher dosage is also associated with more significant side effects.

Other large studies have shown that statin use decreased the risk of heart attack, stroke, peripheral arterial disease, and death in men and women, middle aged and older persons, and people who had not yet had a heart attack as well as those who had survived a significant heart event. With results like these, physician confidence in the use of statins is high. They are generally considered a very cost-effective medication, second only to aspirin, in the prevention of heart attack and stroke.

Types of statins include but are not limited to lovastatin, simvastatin, pravastatin, fluvastatin, and atorvastatin. These are marketed under the brand names Mevacor, Zocor, Pravachol, Lescol, and Lipitor, respectively. Since the body makes more cholesterol at night than during the day, patients are usually directed to take statins in a single dose at the evening meal or bedtime.

Typically, statins impact cholesterol levels the most by about four to six weeks. After about six to eight weeks, your health care provider will retest your cholesterol levels to determine the effectiveness of the therapy and whether the dose requires adjustment.

Most people do not have serious side effects when taking statins; some people may experience constipation, stomach pain, cramps, or gas. These symptoms are usually mild to moderate, however, and go away over time. More serious side effects can result from an increase in liver enzymes that can lead to liver toxicity. Because of this risk, it's important to have your liver function tested periodically while you are on statin therapy. People with active chronic liver disease should not take statins.

ALERT

Certain studies have shown a possible increased risk of amnesia and other memory-related problems while on statins. While this is possibly a rare side effect, more research is required. Since cholesterol is essential to cell membrane structure, scientists suggest that reducing cholesterol may affect neurological functioning.

Another serious side effect comes from statin myopathy. Muscle soreness, pain, and weakness may occur. In extreme cases, muscle cells can break down and release the protein myoglobin into the blood. Myoglobin in the urine can contribute to impaired kidney function, eventually leading to kidney failure. The risk of this occurring increases when statins are taken at high dosages or combined with certain other cholesterol medications. Since statins affect the cell membrane's synthesis of cholesterol, women who are pregnant or planning to become pregnant should absolutely avoid them.

Avoid consuming grapefruit juice, grapefruits, or tangelos (a hybrid grapefruit) when you are taking statins, as these fruits can affect how the drug is metabolized. Grapefruits contain a chemical that affects certain digestive enzymes as drugs are broken down in the intestinal tract and liver. Interestingly, this effect can occur even if you wait twenty-four hours to take the medication. Therefore, if you are taking statins, it is best to avoid grapefruit products entirely.

Bile Acid Sequestrants

Bile acid sequestrants, also referred to as bile acid resins, reduce LDL cholesterol by binding with cholesterol-rich bile acids in the intestines to facilitate their elimination from the body through the stool. Think back to the liver's role in the cholesterol-manufacturing process. The liver uses cholesterol to manufacture bile acids, a digestive enzyme that breaks down fats. Bile acid sequestrants cause the body to eliminate bile acids in the intestines. Since the body needs bile acids to digest fats, the liver must manufacture more bile acids to replace those eliminated by the drug. The liver uses up its available cholesterol to make more acids, thus making less cholesterol available for release into the bloodstream. Bile acid sequestrants can reduce LDL levels 10–20 percent. Bile acid resins, however, can raise triglycerides. Researchers have found a reduction in risk of coronary artery disease through the use of bile acid sequestrants, though this reduction is not nearly as significant as the risk reduction by statins.

Types of bile acid resins include cholestyramine (brand name Prevalite or Questran) and colestipol (Colestid). Cholestyramine and colestipol are often taken as powders that are mixed with water or fruit juice and taken either once or twice a day with meals. Both drugs are also available as tablets.

FACT

Federal government guidelines call for consideration of bile acid sequestrants as LDL-lowering therapy for women with elevated LDL cholesterol who are considering pregnancy, or for combination therapy with statins in people with very high LDL cholesterol levels.

The principal side effects with the use of bile acid resins have to do with digestion. This type of drug can cause a variety of gastrointestinal problems, such as constipation, bloating, fullness, nausea, abdominal pain, and gas. Drinking lots of water and eating high-fiber foods can help with these side effects. Physicians generally do not prescribe bile acid resins to people with a history of constipation problems.

Taking bile acids can also inhibit the absorption of certain nutrients from foods and of other medications. Physicians recommend you take other prescription medications at least one hour before or at least four to six hours after the bile acid sequestrant. They also inhibit the absorption of fat-soluble vitamins from food, namely vitamins A, D, E, and K, so vitamin supplementation may be necessary, especially if taking bile acid sequestrants during pregnancy.

Nicotinic Acid

Nicotinic acid, also known as niacin or vitamin B3, is gaining favor as a way to reduce total blood cholesterol, LDL cholesterol, and triglyceride levels and to elevate HDL levels. At extremely high doses, nicotinic acid raises HDL and transforms small LDL into the less harmful, normal-sized LDL. Niacin therapy moderately reduces LDL levels. Among all the pharmaceutical choices, nicotinic acid is the most effective in raising HDL.

QUESTION

Can you just take high doses of over-the-counter niacin for your high cholesterol?
Self-treatment with niacin is not safe. Since dosage and timing are important, people should not attempt to self-medicate with over-the-counter B3 vitamins. Treatment with this medication should take place only under the recommendation and supervision of a doctor.

Studies demonstrate the power of niacin treatment on lipid disorders. Patients treated with immediate-release niacin have seen their HDL levels increase 15–35 percent, along with a 20–50 percent reduction in triglycerides and a 10–20 percent reduction in LDL cholesterol. Niacin has been shown to help reverse atherosclerosis, therefore likely decreasing the chance of a heart attack or stroke.

Niacin formulations come in three categories: immediate-release, short-term or intermediate release, and sustained or slow-acting release. If you are a candidate for niacin therapy, your physician will determine what formulation suits you. Most physicians start patients on a low dose and work up to a daily dose of 1.5–3 grams. This improves the body's acceptance of the drug.

Another important consideration among different products is the quality of the niacin and the amount the body will absorb. A challenge with many over-the-counter supplements is they are prepared in forms that do not break down easily in the digestive system. They essentially pass through the body, without allowing absorption of any nutrients. Supplements are not regulated by the U.S. Food and Drug Administration and are therefore not guaranteed to provide what is claimed on the labels.

Niaspan, produced by KOS Pharmaceuticals, is specially formulated and packaged in a way that makes it clear how to regulate the levels of niacin in the bloodstream. Nicotinamide is another form of niacin; however, it is not effective in lowering cholesterol levels.

The challenge with niacin treatment is tolerability. Flushing or hot flashes and itching, the result of the opening of blood vessels, are the most common side effects. If you titrate the drugs appropriately, however, the side effects should decrease over time as your body becomes more tolerant of the therapy. Taking niacin during or after meals and additional medications recommended by your physician can also decrease flushing. Taking aspirin thirty minutes prior to niacin has shown to reduce the incidence of flushing by 90 percent.

FACT

Federal government guidelines suggest nicotinic acid as a therapeutic option for higher-risk people, often as combination therapy, or as a single agent if the higher-risk person does not have high LDL levels.

Other side effects include gastrointestinal upset such as nausea, indigestion, gas, vomiting, diarrhea, and even peptic ulcers. More serious risks include liver problems, gout, and high blood sugar. These risks increase as the dosage level is increased. People who take high blood pressure medications also need to exercise caution with niacin therapy. Taking niacin can amplify the effects of blood pressure medications. People with diabetes typically do not receive niacin therapy because of its effect on blood sugar.

Fibrates

Physicians prescribe fibrates, or fibric acid derivatives, primarily to reduce triglycerides but also to increase HDL cholesterol. Fibrates, however, do not lower LDL cholesterol. Since LDL reduction is usually the primary target of therapy, fibrates are not typically physicians' drug of choice for individuals with elevated cholesterol levels. You should, however, evaluate the relevance of fibrate therapy to your individual case, since it is the drug of choice to reduce the most harmful small, dense LDL particles.

Fibrate therapy is a treatment option for people with coronary artery disease who have low LDL but who still have unhealthy triglyceride levels. Physicians may prescribe fibrates along with statins for people who have both high levels of LDL and unhealthy triglyceride levels.

Studies show that fibrates can reduce triglycerides by as much as 20–50 percent and can increase HDL by 10–15 percent. According to federal government guidelines, physicians can prescribe fibrates to people with very high triglycerides to reduce risk of acute pancreatitis, as extremely high triglyceride levels can occasionally cause inflammation of the pancreas.

ALERT

Taking fibrates can increase the effect of blood-thinning medications. If you are taking both fibrates and blood thinners, work closely with your physician to monitor the effect of the fibrates.

Gemfibrozil and fenofibrate are types of fibrates, known by the brand names Lopid and Tricor. Clofibrate is the third fibrate available in the United States. People on fibrate therapy typically take a dose twice daily, usually thirty minutes before their morning and evening meals.

Most people do not suffer any adverse side effects from fibrate therapy. Some people, however, do experience gastrointestinal problems or headache, dizziness, blurred vision, runny nose, fatigue, or flushing. For some people, fibrates increase the chances of developing gallstones. Combining statins with fibrates may increase muscle cell breakdown or rhabdomyolysis, which can potentially also harm the kidneys, which receive the products of the muscle breakdown. Tell your health care provider right away about any side effects, particularly if you experience muscle or joint pain or weakness.

Blood Pressure Drugs

Blood pressure is the longest and best known of the medically treatable risk factors, while being the most easily and commonly tested. Because of this, many classes of medications have been researched and tested for years, and their efficacy has been proven in decreasing the chance of developing some of the complications of cardiovascular disease.

Beta-Blockers

Beta-blockers, such as Atenolol, Propanolol, and Metoprolol, function by blocking so-called beta receptors on the heart. These receptors control the rate of the heart's contractions and the strength of each contraction. By slowing the rate and strength of the contractions, blood is pumped less forcefully in the body. Because blood is pumped less forcefully, less pressure is exerted by the blood on blood vessel walls. In other words, blood pressure is reduced.

Because the heart is slowed and blood is pumped less forcefully, exercise tolerance is significantly reduced, a common side effect of beta-blockers. Also, because there is less blood pumped to organs like the brain, you can develop significant lightheadedness, a known, common complication of beta-blockers. As beta-blockers slow the pacemaker of the heart, they can cause heart blocks, where the heart does not pump as often as it should.

Beta-receptors exist on other organs of the body, causing other side effects. Beta-receptors open up the lungs. Therefore, blocking of beta-receptors can worsen conditions such as asthma or emphysema. To combat this problem, newer beta-blockers more specific to heart receptors have been developed, such as metoprolol and atenolol.

Blocking beta-receptors may also make it harder for diabetics to control their blood sugars as well as to feel the symptoms of hypoglycemia or low blood sugar, making it harder to correct immediately. Many other organs have beta-receptors, causing other side effects such as nightmares and confusion. Beta-blockers can also worsen HDL.

Despite worsening other risk factors, beta-blockers have been repeatedly shown to reduce mortality from many cardiovascular diseases. As they can worsen other risk factors and require closer monitoring and treatment of those factors, lifestyle modifications are still the first choice.

Calcium-Channel Blockers

Calcium-channel blockers, such as nifedipine (or Norvasc), decrease high blood pressure by blocking calcium-channel depolarization in the heart and blood vessels. In your heart, the cells function by opening pathways for calcium to get in the cells, changing the electricity of the cell so that a signal is transmitted. By blocking these channels and therefore this signal, the heart's pacemaker fires slower and the heart does not contract as strongly. The mechanism of calcium-channel blockers is similar to beta-blockers in reducing high blood pressure; also, similarly, a dangerous side effect is heartbeat blockade, or not pumping enough blood to meet the demands of the brain or exercising tissues.

ESSENTIAL

While beta-blockers and calcium-channel blockers reduce the workload of the heart, they also make it harder for the heart to meet the demands of exercising. When you cannot exercise it can worsen your risk factors for heart disease. While the medications have shown to be effective, the ideal is to try to prevent or treat high blood pressure without medication.

Unlike beta-blockers, calcium-channel blockers used to treat hypertension have more of an effect on blood vessels as well, causing them to dilate and therefore reducing the pressure blood and vessels exert on each other. Though there exists calcium-channel blockers that are more selective of the heart, like beta-blockers, because of these dilating effects, nifedipine is the most commonly used calcium-channel blocker to treat high blood pressure.

Nifedipine can cause constipation due to blocking calcium channels in the gut, redness in the face from blood vessel dilation, and fluid buildup in the legs.

ACE Inhibitors/ARBs

ACE or Angiotensin-Converting Enzyme inhibitors, rather than working on the heart, work on the kidney's regulation of blood pressure. Some examples include Captopril, Enalapril, and Lisinopril. The kidney helps regulate blood pressure, which is why when risk factors such as hypertension and diabetes that can harm the kidneys go unchecked, there can be even more issues with blood pressure.

The kidneys have sensors that detect the pressure of blood on the kidney. In response to how much pressure the kidneys receive, they release a chemical called renin, which gets converted to angiotensin. Angiotensin then gets converted by Angiotensin-Converting Enzyme in the lungs and kidneys to a chemical that raises blood pressure in several ways. One of these ways is increasing the reabsorption of salt by the kidneys. Remember, through osmosis, where salt goes water follows, causing more fluid retention in the body, which then increases blood pressure. In addition, blood vessels constrict more tightly, which also raises blood pressure. By blocking the formation of this chemical, these effects do not occur, and blood pressure is reduced.

As with all blood pressure lowering medicines, these can cause dizziness and lightheadedness. In addition, because of their effects on lungs and kidneys, they can cause chronic cough and kidney failure. Also, with the effects on the reabsorption of fluid and the kidneys' management of electrolytes, they can cause low sodium and high potassium.

Angiotensin-Receptor Blockers or ARBs such as Losartan (or Cozaar), rather than inhibiting the formation of the chemical that causes all the effects that raise blood pressure, work by blocking the receptors that receive that chemical. Because of this bypass mechanism, they do not have all of the side effects of ACE-Inhibitors such as a cough, and are intended for those who cannot tolerate ACE-Inhibitors.

Diuretics

Diuretics represent several classes of medicine that work by promoting increased urination. Less fluid in the body results in less pressure on blood vessel walls by blood, thereby lowering blood pressure.

The two most common diuretics are Furosemide (or Lasix) and Hydrochlorothiazide. These act on receptors in the kidney that block the reabsorption of certain electrolytes. As we discussed with ACE-Inhibitors, as more electrolytes are urinated out, fluid follows.

Obvious side effects of these medications are dehydration and abnormalities in the electrolytes such as potassium, sodium, and calcium. The dehydration and electrolyte abnormalities can cause disturbances in muscles and nerves causing symptoms that range from relatively minor, such as muscle cramping, to very severe, such as muscle breakdown and seizures.

In addition, diuretics can raise the amount of uric acid in your body, the chemical responsible for most cases of gout. Therefore, diuretics should be avoided in those with a history of gout. Diuretics should also not be taken by those with sulfa allergies.

FACT

Many other medications exist to treat high blood pressure, but beta-blockers, calcium-channel blockers, ACE-Inhibitors, and diuretics are by far the most commonly used. If you are prescribed a different medication, it is likely for reasons worth inquiring about.

Diabetes Drugs

In addition to cardiovascular disease, diabetes has many other devastating effects on the body. It hurts the body's ability to heal, affects sensation in the extremities, can cause kidney failure, and can worsen vision. These effects can be minimized with the strict control of blood sugar through dietary modification and medication.

Insulin

For years, insulin was the only medication to treat diabetes. As you recall, diabetes can either be due to a lack of insulin in type 1 diabetes or to a resistance to insulin in type 2 diabetes. Insulin is still the treatment of choice for type 1 diabetes, due to a need to replace the body's inability to produce insulin.

Over the years, many types of insulin have been developed, through the recombination of the DNA sequences that create the insulin protein. The main difference between these different types of insulin is their duration of action.

The most commonly used insulins are Lispro, also known as regular insulin, and NPH. Lispro is a short-acting insulin, typically taken after meals to combat the blood sugar rises that come after meals. NPH is an intermediate-acting insulin that is taken to lower blood sugars over the course of a day or night. Most insulin-dependent diabetics will take some combination of both.

All insulins are delivered by injection, as ingestion would cause the breakdown of the insulin protein in the gut. Some people use insulin pumps, worn twenty-four hours a day, that steadily inject the necessary amount of insulin into the body.

The main side effect of insulin is low blood sugar. Studies have repeatedly confirmed that the stricter you are able to control your blood sugar, the less chance you have to develop some of the complications of diabetes, including heart disease.

Metformin

For type 2 diabetes, though, because the body has developed a resistance to insulin, other medicines are used as well. This is not to say insulin is not used, as although there is a resistance to insulin, it still has some efficacy. These other medicines, known as oral hypoglycemics, can also be used. Unlike insulin, they're able to be swallowed as a pill without losing their function. The most commonly used oral hypoglycemic is metformin, or Glucophage. Metformin is considered the first-line choice because it causes less severe hypoglycemia than some of the other oral hypoglycemics. The mechanism of metformin is not completely understood, but it is believed that parts of its effect comes from both reducing the formation of sugar in the blood from stored sugar in the liver and promoting the storage of blood sugar into cells, thereby mimicking the effect of insulin.

ESSENTIAL

Because of the risk of hypoglycemia from insulin and oral hypoglycemics, diabetics on medications must eat regular meals to maintain their blood sugar, otherwise they could experience a severe hypoglycemic reaction, which could be as serious as paralysis or death.

The most common side effect of metformin is diarrhea and heartburn. The most serious side effect is increased acid in those with impaired kidney function. Because kidney problems are common in diabetics, it is very important that kidney function be checked before starting this medication.

Glitazones

Glitazones such as Actos and Avandia act by decreasing the body's resistance to insulin. The insulin the body is already making can therefore have more of an effect again, improving regulation of blood sugar, and over the long term, decreasing the complications of diabetes.

The main side effects of these medications are water retention. If the water retention is severe enough, it can exacerbate congestive heart failure. These medications should therefore be used with caution in those already with a history of heart failure. As with almost all diabetes medications, the most common serious side effect is hypoglycemia, especially when used with other diabetes medications.

In recent studies, Avandia has been shown to actually increase the risk of cardiac events by mechanisms that are not fully understood, and the drug is therefore no longer in favor. Actos, on the other hand, has been shown to decrease cardiovascular events of almost every nature and is now considered first line among glitazone medications.

Sulfonylureas

Sulfonylureas such as glipizide and glyburide act by increasing the release of insulin from the pancreas. In other words, when the body is resistant to the amount of insulin it is currently making, these medications act by releasing more in an attempt to overcome that resistance. These make them the most prone to hypoglycemia among the oral hypoglycemics, since they actually stimulate the release of more insulin. They are also known to cause stomach pain and headaches.

Sulfonylureas should not be used in those with sulfa allergies. These medications are also known to be teratogenic, or to cause birth defects, so should be avoided in pregnant women. They are also known to cause increased hypoglycemia in those with kidney and liver failure and should not be used for those patients. In general, insulin is recommended as the primary treatment for any sort of diabetes in pregnant women and those with kidney and liver failure, though more research is suggesting certain oral hypoglycemics may be useful. Though these medications have been shown to reduce high blood sugar, they have yet to be shown to decrease cardiovascular complications. In fact, some research has suggested that they increase the risk of certain cardiovascular diseases; therefore, these medications carry an FDA-required warning regarding an increased risk of cardiovascular death.

ESSENTIAL

Despite many medications in existence that should, in theory, reduce the complications of cardiovascular disease, many of these medications have yet to show a significant reduction in cardiovascular events—such as sulfonylureas—and some show more cardiovascular events—such as Avandia. Lifestyle modification, on the other hand, consistently shows improved outcomes.

Tips for Following Your Medication Program

Following your doctor's recommendations makes sense. Your health care provider is a trained professional who has taken time and effort to develop a program of therapy to support your well-being. Studies show that many patients do not follow medical advice. If you have taken the time to pursue a program, make the best of this support and follow your medication program. The following tips can help you.

FACT

According to the American Heart Association, 10 percent of all hospital admissions are patients who did not take their medications according to the instructions. The average stay in American hospitals due to medical noncompliance is 4.2 days. More than half of all Americans with chronic diseases do not follow their physician's medication and lifestyle instructions.

One of the most important things you can do to help you to stay on your medication program is to understand exactly what type of medication you are taking and why it is best for a person in your condition. This requires you to take some initiative to educate yourself about your lipid profile, your cholesterol goals, and your dosage schedule. Ask your health care provider the following questions:

- What is my goal of therapy?
- What type of medication am I taking?
- Why is that medication best for a person in my condition?
- Are there any food/drug combinations I should avoid?
- When should I take the medicine and should I take it with, before, or after meals?
- What should I do if I forget to take a dose?
- What are the side effects of the medication and when should I contact a health care provider?
- Who should I contact, and how, in case I have negative side effects?

Consistency is essential to getting the most out of your therapeutic program. Do not change your dosage amount or schedule or quit taking prescription medications without consulting your physician. If you have a hard time with consistency, try some of the following tips:

- Take your medicine at the same time each day.
- Take your medicine when you perform a specific daily act, such as before you brush your teeth.
- Set your watch alarm as a pill reminder.
- Write yourself a note in a prominent place.
- Use a pillbox that holds each day's prescriptions in their respective compartments in a place where you will not forget to take them at the appropriate time.
- Write prescription renewal notes in your calendar to remind you before prescriptions run out.

If none of these tips help, consult with your pharmacist for more ideas. Work together with your health care provider as a team. Observe your reactions to the medication. Take notes, and report everything back to your physician. Keep your follow-up appointments so you can discuss how things are going. Bring your observation notes to your appointment to remind you of things you may easily forget. Bring your prescription bottles as well. Follow your progress from visit to visit—record data in a log or notebook. If you have questions, ask them: Communication is critical to getting the best health care.

CHAPTER 8

Creating Your Healthy Lifestyle

According to the Centers for Disease Control and Prevention, about half of all deaths in the United States are linked to behaviors that are changeable. In other words, most people can do simple things to prolong their lives. Perhaps even more important, you can add to your quality of life by avoiding heart attacks or strokes. By making healthy choices, you will live longer, enjoy a higher quality of life, feel better about yourself, have more energy, and reduce your risks of disease and disability.

The Power to Create Health

You've learned about the risk factors. You've learned that you can improve your overall health. All this knowledge is meaningless if not applied to improve your life or the lives of others. The purpose of this chapter is to give you insight into what it means to create a healthy standard of living. This means understanding not only the individual pieces of the puzzle—like eating better or exercising more—but also how to fit them all together over a lifetime. Regardless of how difficult the challenge of changing your life, the rewards of simple healthy living are worth the commitment and effort.

ALERT

In today's environment, if you don't have an aggressive strategy for eating whole foods and incorporating physical activities, it is easy to gain weight. Most easy-access foods are loaded with salt, fat, sugar, and other unhealthy substances. It's also much easier not to put any effort into exercise. But if you go through life passively and do what is easiest and most convenient, your choices are likely to lead to premature death and disability.

What Science Can Teach Us

The great benefit of being alive today is that scientific research provides an almost complete picture of the mechanisms behind atherosclerosis and heart disease. In the process of unraveling how the physical system develops disease, even more insight is gained into how to prevent, or at least deter, the disease processes.

What You Can Do

What science cannot change is that *you* are the bottom line. Just as money cannot buy happiness, it cannot buy health. Money can buy access to the best health care providers, to all the procedures and drugs that are available, and to minimally processed whole foods, but even the wealthiest people cannot buy good health. Health must be created through active effort.

The World Health Organization defines health as "a state of complete physical, social, and mental well-being, not merely the absence of disease or infirmity." This definition of health is very expansive. It supposes an optimal condition of being, rather than a minimal state of being disease free. So instead of putting your focus on how to stop disease, consider shifting your focus to how to create optimal health. You have the power to achieve it. All you need is the knowledge, which this book can help provide, and the motivation, which comes from deep within yourself.

The Hazards of Modern Living

One of the greatest ironies of modern living is that it is actually much easier to survive in a manner that contributes to poor health and chronic disease than it is to live a life of vibrant, vital health. The reasons for this are many and complex. Some of the factors of modern convenience are closely intertwined with the leading risk factors for heart disease.

Poor Eating Habits

The foods that are easiest to obtain and most plentiful are fast, high-fat, high-sugar, calorie-rich, highly refined processed foods. These foods are often nutrient poor, yet cheap and effortless to find. It takes more time and dedication to find and prepare natural, whole foods. Fortunately, more and more grocery stores and restaurants offering healthy fare are opening everywhere, but healthy living still takes effort. But the rewards of eating such health-enhancing foods are clear: You will live longer and feel better.

What you eat has a powerful influence over your blood pressure, blood sugar, and cholesterol. Research supports that eating a primarily plant-based diet that consists of a large proportion of minimally processed (or whole) grains, vegetables, and fruits is essential to support optimal health.

Lack of Exercise and Excess Weight

Modern innovations have created so many labor-saving devices that the requirement to move is almost obsolete: you can drive to work or to run errands; sit in a chair to perform your job; shop and play games on your computer; use elevators and escalators to transport your body; and even use remote-control devices to operate the appliances in your home. Physical education is no longer a required daily curriculum for many children, and stationary, technology-driven activities are often childrens' choice for play instead of physical outdoor games. This is not good for health. To create optimum health, the human body needs physical activity.

All of this technology means that things people used to take for granted, such as walking around each day to complete tasks or even to have fun and play, are no longer an essential part of modern lives. Instead, people need to plan for movement. They need to brainstorm strategies to stay active. All of this inactivity has contributed to weight gain. When the inactivity is combined with easy-to-grab calorie-rich foods, even more weight gain is the result.

Exposure to Toxins

Another aspect of modern living that makes it difficult to support health is that you are exposed to environmental toxins, including numerous carcinogens. Cigarette smoke, air pollution, and other harmful chemicals in the air, water, and food supply undermine people's well-being. Scientific studies have proved them harmful to both human health and to the environment.

ALERT

Chemicals and other toxins in the water, air, buildings, and food supply are impossible to avoid completely. Although you cannot totally control the environment you live in, you can do your part to minimize dangerous exposures, whether not smoking, filtering water, or eating whole foods.

Mental Stress

One of the most prominent features of modern living is the difficulty of escaping the mental stresses of daily life. Technology continues to drive the pace of work and living to faster and faster speeds. The cost of living, the pressure of competition for material wealth, and the challenge of balancing family, professional, and community ties all contribute to increasing daily pressures. Finding time to relax, unwind, and savor simple pleasures becomes a rare treat and often requires effort in itself.

One of the greatest dangers of stress is the damage it does to your body. Stress releases the chemical cortisol. Cortisol creates free radicals, which contribute to plaque formation. Stress also raises your blood pressure, blood sugar, and worsens your cholesterol profile, creating even more risk for a stroke or a heart attack.

The Process of Change

As you get ready to embark on your own path toward healthful living, it is useful to learn not only what to change, but how to change it. Behavioral-medicine researchers constantly examine how to support the process of change. Most people know they should eat more fruits and vegetables, exercise more regularly, decrease stress, and not smoke, so the question for scientists becomes, "Why aren't more people doing it?" Researchers realize that changing behaviors is a very difficult task, and they seek to understand how to improve the process to maximize people's odds of success.

Not all people follow a linear path on the road to change. For example, a person may progress to the action stage and then return to the contemplation stage. What is important is that you continue to try—don't let your setbacks become permanent.

A leading psychological model for behavioral change divides the course of action into five stages of readiness that are very useful for analysis. Understanding this progression can help you find success in achieving your goal of living a healthier lifestyle. The five stages include precontemplation, contemplation, preparation, action, and maintenance.

These phases are meant to describe the process of becoming more ready for change. If the process is cultivated in that order—motivation first, action second—the odds of ultimate success in achieving lifestyle changes are much higher. Action without motivation may get things started, but it is simply not sustainable.

Precontemplation

Congratulations! Anyone who is reading this book has already progressed beyond the precontemplation stage. A person in the precontemplation stage is not making any behavioral changes and does not intend to make any changes. They are not motivated and do not have the tools and information necessary to make a positive change. It is easier to stay in their situation and even risk poor health and a shorter life than it is to make any changes. You may have friends or loved ones who are at this level.

Contemplation

In the contemplation stage, you know it is better to live a healthier lifestyle. Although you are thinking about it, you haven't taken any action toward making this change a reality. During this stage, you are engaged in information gathering and weighing the pros and cons of taking any action. You haven't made any commitment to change, you are just thinking about it. This, however, is a very important stage. If you feel you are in this stage, you are doing exactly the right thing by reading and learning more about the benefits of making positive modifications toward a healthier lifestyle.

QUESTION

How can I help friends or loved ones who are in the contemplation stage?
The best way to provide support is to share information about specific benefits that come with adopting healthier behaviors. For example, tell them that a person who starts a moderate exercise program will sleep better at night and have more energy during the day. These are usually benefits everyone can relate to and want to enjoy.

Preparation

People who are in the preparation stage have already started taking small steps toward acquiring new, healthy habits. For example, if you plan more physical pursuits, you have gone out and bought a new pair of walking shoes. Or, if you want to eat more healthfully, you have purchased a book such as this one, full of heart-healthy recipes and tips for incorporating better snacking habits.

To help keep yourself motivated, keep visual cues and props in obvious places. For example, post pictures of fruits, vegetables, whole grains, or fit and healthy role models on the refrigerator. Keep workout equipment such as shoes both at home and in the office. Persist in learning about all the benefits available from eating nutritious foods, staying active, managing stress, and feeling your best.

Action

In the action stage, things start to get exciting. This is the first six-month period of starting up a new exercise program, following a new eating pattern, or of integrating new methods of relaxation into your day. Studies show that it typically takes two months to develop a new habit and that as many as 50 percent of people who start a new program drop out within the first six months. Strategies to make it through the first six months include eliciting support from friends, family, and coworkers, and keeping useful reminders in places that you look frequently. The most important thing is using your motivation and contemplation to make sure you create the time and organize your life so you can sustain your newly developed habits.

Maintenance

The ideal conclusion to a concentrated effort in making a behavioral change is to reach the maintenance phase. In the example of incorporating regular activity, you get to the maintenance phase when you have exercised regularly for at least six months. By this point, you get used to the time and ways you exercise. Sustaining the behavior becomes much easier and self-motivating, because it is easy to feel the benefits and rewards of the healthy activity.

This does not mean it does not require effort to sustain the activity, so do not let your guard down. As always, being healthy will take effort and motivation. It's important to incorporate fun and different activities to keep motivation levels high, and the longer the behavior is continued the less likely you are to drop it.

Dealing with Relapse

As the saying goes, humans are creatures of habit. Change is not easy. Relapsing is a normal part of the process. In fact, studies show that people who ultimately succeed in quitting smoking have usually tried to quit at least three times.

If you relapse, approach the process of change as a learning experience. With every step forward, figure out what worked. With every step backward, rather than beating yourself up, try to determine why that backward step occurred. If you approach transformation of your habits as a journey and self-learning adventure, you are likely to find more success. Forgive yourself and keep on going.

ESSENTIAL

Your new health practices, such as eating a piece of fruit for breakfast or completing a set of pushups in the morning, are not burdensome "problems" or "prescriptive medicines." View them as solutions that will improve your life, not another duty to add to your list of chores. Rather than thinking about the energy it's taking, think about the energy you are gaining.

Find ways to incorporate healthy habits that work for you so that you will continue to do them. For example, if you don't care for raisins, don't plan to eat them on your oatmeal every morning for breakfast. Instead, find something that you like to eat that is also good for you and plan to include more of it in your diet. Perhaps you enjoy blackberries or smoothies. Perhaps you enjoy swimming more than running. Maybe even a nicotine patch is enough to keep you from smoking—even that is a healthier alternative.

If you find that you need someone to help keep you accountable with your diet or in a regular exercise program, consult a registered dietitian or hire a personal trainer to work with on a regular basis. Enlist your friends and family. One of the best sources of motivation for anyone is not wanting to let others down, even more than not wanting to let yourself down. Find solutions that work and make you feel good about you.

Believe in Yourself

Another important concept researchers have determined is fundamental to successful change is how much you believe in your own ability to achieve it. Self-confidence is important; the more you believe you can achieve success, the more likely you are to find it. In contrast, if you see yourself as a person who simply can't eat nutritious foods or possibly find time to move around more during the day, then it will come true for you.

ALERT

Studies show that if you engage in behaviors that promote health, you can add as much as twenty years to the length of your life. This holds true even if you start incorporating more healthy behaviors at the age of fifty.

Changing your thoughts, like anything else, requires active effort. It may mean paying more attention to your thoughts in general and, when you notice a negative one, escaping that thought pattern. You might distract yourself with other more positive thoughts or even pinch yourself to condition yourself away from self-defeating thinking. As with contemplation and motivation, you may find it possible to change your thoughts for the better by changing your environment with positive photos, exercise equipment, and the right foods.

Identify Your Priorities

Here's an interesting exercise to help you get in touch with what really matters in your life. Take a few moments to write down the top five things that are important to you. Examples of items you may want to include are your family, health, community, profession, a hobby, political causes, or volunteer work. Then, on the same piece of paper, list the top five activities that take up most of your time in an average day. Note the percentage of your waking time that they require.

Take a moment to compare how you spend your time each day with what you value most in your life. Have you found a good match? Or have you realized that you are neglecting some things that are very important to you? Once you increase your awareness of the way you are spending your time versus the way you want to spend your time, you can start making a difference. As you bring your unconscious habits and behavior patterns out into the open, you can begin to realistically assess small steps you can take toward your new goals.

For example, if you realize that you are spending three hours each day watching television and no time walking or participating in any other type of moderate physical activity, you can see that there is some time in your day that you can carve out to use for exercising. Or consider ways to do some exercises as you watch your favorite programs.

How can understanding your risk factors help with spending more time on your priorities? With your risk factors under control, and by following a sensible diet and exercise program, you'll have more energy, more time for activities, and a longer life to achieve your goals.

You May Have Just Saved a Life—Yours

Last, but certainly not least, remember to reward yourself for your good behavior. For example, promise yourself that if you stick to your new eating plan or exercise schedule for four consecutive weeks, (or, ideally, six months) you will reward yourself with a nice massage or buy yourself some new exercise clothes. Of course, the greatest reward will be how your new health will benefit you and your loved ones.

Living in a time when you can better understand your health and strive to optimize it is truly a privilege. When you move about, enjoy the sensation of your muscles in action. As you eat a dish of fresh foods, savor the flavors, colors, aroma, and textures that whole foods add to your dining pleasure. And as you feel stronger, more energetic, and simply more alive, know that it is the direct result of your efforts to create a healthy life. You can do it—just keep believing in yourself and in your worth, because you *are* worth it.

CHAPTER 9

Strategies for Heart-Healthy Eating

Knowing what foods are good for you is only half the story; figuring out how to eat them regularly is the challenging part. Changing your routine is never easy, but you can do it if you keep taking small, steady steps. The tips in this chapter will help you move toward a healthier pattern of eating. Once you start feeling the benefits of enjoying more fresh, wholesome foods, your new habits will become self-reinforcing. Enjoy the process as you travel toward a healthier you.

Eat Healthful Plant-Based Foods

A nutritious diet is key to creating long-term health. Poor nutrition is one of the leading causes of heart disease. The old adage "You are what you eat" is actually quite true. Your body derives its nutrients, its building blocks for cellular repair and growth, and its fuel for all activities directly from the food you consume.

The connection between food and your blood-cholesterol levels is direct and powerful. Overconsumption of saturated fats, trans fats, simple sugars, and cholesterol-rich foods leads to overproduction of LDL cholesterol in the liver and the release of excess amounts of triglycerides into the bloodstream. Saturated fats and cholesterol are present only in animal foods. Trans fats are present only in processed, commercial foods.

When you alter your eating habits to include more plant-based foods and fewer animal-based and processed foods, you take a powerful step toward improving the health of your bloodstream. Studies have shown that nutritional factors alone can reduce LDL by as much as 60 percent in individuals with high levels of cholesterol. This change is far more powerful than the best prescription medications. Another significant difference is that improvements in nutrition do not have the same risk of adverse side effects as taking a long-term prescriptive drug. In fact, the main side effects of eating healthier are more energy, weight loss, a clearer mind, and more radiant skin. Lastly, eating healthier is much more affordable than medications or other more invasive treatments for heart attacks and strokes.

Numerous nutritional studies demonstrate that plant-based foods enhance your health, particularly cardiovascular health. Humans cannot exist without plant foods. While it is possible to live healthfully over a lifetime without any consumption of meat, it is not possible to survive without eating plant-based foods.

Moving Away from Meats and Animal Fats

Although researchers have determined that a varied diet of whole fresh foods is the most beneficial to health, you can still enjoy meat as part of a heart-healthy diet; you just need to use it carefully. What you need to focus on is creating dishes from lean cuts of meats and enjoying meats as more of a side dish than a main course. Purchase meats from animals fed grass diets, also called free range, rather than animal fats and animal by-products.

If you eat a typical fast-food diet, it is challenging to convert to a diet of whole fresh foods. The rest of this chapter will provide you with specific strategies for making this transition as smooth as possible. What you eat affects your life in a very intimate way. You need to be able to enjoy your meals and snacks and not feel deprived or punished. Take the time that you need to incorporate healthier foods that you enjoy in order to create lasting changes.

Reducing Saturated Fat in Meats

Eating saturated fats increases the amounts of harmful LDL cholesterol. At the same time, minimizing or avoiding these foods completely in your diet can help to lower harmful LDL levels and reduce your risk of heart disease.

When you prepare meats, try to do so in a manner that reduces rather than increases the amount of fat. For example, baste with wines or marinades and season with herbs; grill or broil meats instead of frying or breading; sauté or brown meats in pans sprayed with vegetable oils. If you are adding meat to other dishes, such as spaghetti, brown it first and pour off the fat before you add it to the sauce. Here are some more preparation tips to reduce saturated fats in meats:

- Trim excess fat from meats.
- Purchase lean meats. For beef, aim for 96 percent lean; for chicken, 99 percent lean.
- Avoid purchasing meats that are marbled with fat.
- Remove skin from poultry.
- Broil, grill, roast, or bake meats on racks that allow fats to drain off.
- Skim fats from tops of stews or casseroles.
- Limit or avoid organ meats, such as livers, brains, sweetbreads, and kidneys.
- Limit or avoid processed meats, such as lunchmeat, salami, bologna, pepperoni, or sausage.
- Serve smaller portions of meats.
- Try substituting lean ground turkey or chicken for beef and pork.

These preparation tips will not only reduce the harmful saturated fats in your diet, they will also lower the total fat that you consume, which will help you manage your weight successfully.

ALERT

Cows are naturally grass-eating animals. Meat from grass-fed cattle has about one-half to one-third the fat as meat from grain-fed cattle. Grass-fed beef is lower in calories and higher in vitamin E, omega-3 fatty acids, and conjugated linoleic acid, another health-enhancing fatty acid.

Lowering Saturated Fats from Dairy Products

While dairy products are a valuable source of calcium and protein, they are not the only sources of these important nutrients. Keep in mind that eating lots of full-fat dairy products increases the levels of saturated fat in your diet, which directly increases your levels of LDL. You can still enjoy dairy foods; simply choose low-fat or nonfat versions to promote health, and choose milk from dairy cows that have been fed grass diets.

Cheese, in particular, is a very high-fat food, even higher than beef. While you may choose an occasional treat of creamy cheeses, indulging in them regularly will increase your risk of heart disease. Here are some practical tips for lowering the amount of saturated dairy fat in your diet:

- Choose ½ percent, 1 percent, or, ideally, nonfat milk preferably from grass-fed cows.
- Select nonfat or at least low-fat yogurt, sour cream, and cottage and cream cheese.
- Use lower fat cheeses for cooking, such as part-skim mozzarella, ricotta, or Parmesan.
- Enjoy rich, creamy, and hard cheeses on special occasions, not daily.
- Limit the use of butter, and use it sparingly.

Check that dairy products come from cows fed grasses and grains rather than meat by-products. Look for other sources of calcium in your diet. Vegetables such as broccoli, chard, greens, and artichokes are all great sources of dietary calcium, as are calcium-fortified orange juice, some whole-grain cereals, and even vitamins. Check the labels.

Avoiding Trans Fats

Keep in mind that there is no level of consumption of trans fats that is not harmful to health. These fats increase your LDL cholesterol and decrease your HDL cholesterol levels. Trans fats are found naturally in some dairy and meat products, but most trans fats in the food supply are created artificially through a process called hydrogenation. This converts a liquid fat to a solid.

QUESTION

Why do food manufacturers use hydrogenation?
The benefits to food manufacturers of converting vegetable oils to a solid state is that it gives form to otherwise shapeless foods for easier consumption by hand. The process preserves products and extends the shelf life, and it adds flavor.

Trans fats are abundant in processed foods such as cereals, chips, crackers, stick margarine, shortening, lard, and fried fast foods. Remember that trans fats are sometimes manufactured from vegetable oils, so simply because a food manufacturer indicates that something is prepared with vegetable oil does not mean it is trans-fat free. Also remember that a small serving of any food can contain up to 0.49 grams of trans fat while still reporting 0 grams on the food label.

When reading food labels on items, look for ingredients such as hydrogenated or partially hydrogenated oils, even if they state 0 grams of trans fat. If they are listed, try to avoid using these foods. If you must buy a product with such an ingredient, ensure that the hydrogenated ingredient appears at the end of the ingredient list, indicating that it is present in very low quantities. The goal is to live a trans fat-free life.

You can take the following positive steps to reduce the amounts you consume:

- Avoid or reduce intake of commercially prepared baked goods such as cakes and cookies, snack foods, processed foods, and fast foods.

- Select liquid vegetable oils that contain no trans fats.
- Read margarine labels carefully, and avoid those that contain hydrogenated oils.
- Avoid cooking with lard, shortening, or stick margarine; use vegetable sprays or tub margarine made without trans fats.

Reduce Intake of Dietary Cholesterol

Dietary cholesterol does not elevate blood-cholesterol levels as much as saturated fat. For most people, excess dietary cholesterol is not an issue. The largest source of dietary cholesterol in America is eggs. Studies show that in healthy individuals, consuming one egg per day did not lead to elevated cholesterol levels. If, however, you think that you may be overeating cholesterol, here are some tips on how to reduce your dietary intake:

- Eat egg whites instead of whole eggs.
- Purchase eggs from chickens raised on a vegetarian diet rather than animal fats and animal by-products.
- Read egg-carton labels and compare brands to purchase the most nutritious eggs.
- Limit intake of shellfish high in cholesterol, such as shrimp, abalone, crayfish, and squid. (Other forms of shellfish are not excessively high in cholesterol and can provide valuable nutrients.)

Increasing Vegetables and Fruits

As you reduce the amount of meat you consume, gradually increase the amount of vegetables in your diet. Over time, your taste buds will evolve, and you will enjoy more of the subtle flavors of vegetables and fruits. Your meals will be equally tasty but more colorful and will include more fiber and plant-based nutrients. This reduces not only your risk of cardiovascular disease, but also type 2 diabetes and certain types of cancer.

Try to incorporate fruits or vegetables in every meal and as snacks. Reduce the amount of meat or chicken in typical combination dishes. For example, in spaghetti, reduce the amount of beef or substitute ground turkey. Then increase the vegetable content in your sauces by adding more mushrooms, green peppers, celery, and carrots.

Here are some more tips on how to include more vegetables in your daily diet:

- At breakfast, slice half a banana or toss some berries or raisins on your cereal.
- Add frozen fruits such as berries or peaches to hot cereals.
- At meals, serve larger portions of vegetables, or prepare multiple vegetable dishes and have meat as a side dish.
- Prepare meats with fruit toppings or marinades instead of butter.
- Enjoy fruit-based desserts such as poached pears, baked apples, or fresh-fruit sorbets.
- Buy packaged, prewashed, and sliced veggies to pack as snacks or to eat at lunch.
- Eat fresh whole fruits that are in season as snacks with meals or between them.
- Add vegetables such as peas or beans into rice or pasta dishes.
- Incorporate multiple vegetables into salads in addition to lettuce.
- Enjoy a smoothie made with fruits or vegetables as a beverage.

Keep in mind that all these fruits and vegetables add up to less weight, less disease, less disability, more energy, and a healthy, glowing appearance.

ESSENTIAL

Fruits and vegetables are a great source of fiber. Soluble fiber that's part of a healthy diet can reduce blood-cholesterol levels and the amount of calories you absorb. Some fruits and vegetables that contain soluble fiber, in addition to numerous other beneficial nutrients, include apples with peels, oranges, figs, prunes, peas, broccoli, and carrots.

Enjoying Whole Grains

Whole-grain foods are minimally processed and therefore rich in vitamins, minerals, and fiber. Grains include whole wheat, brown rice, barley, rye, oatmeal, and corn. Whole grains provide complex carbohydrates that are essential for energy and vitamins A and E, magnesium, calcium, and other important nutrients. These fiber-rich foods contain both soluble and insoluble fiber, but they mostly contain insoluble fiber, which aids digestion, keeps your colon healthy, and makes you feel full, helping with weight management. Processed grains, in contrast, are simple carbohydrates and have lost many of the nutrients and the fiber.

Oatmeal that contains oat bran is a rich source of soluble fiber that can help lower cholesterol levels. Food manufacturers often remove the oat bran in the instant-cook varieties. Be sure to purchase whole oats or oat bran to obtain the cholesterol-lowering results.

Ideally, you should eat six servings of grains per day. Here are some tips to add more whole grains into your daily diet:

- Include a grain-based food at every meal.
- Make sure the food is labeled "whole" on the front and in the ingredients list.
- Try whole-grain rolls, breadsticks, crackers, and muffins for snacks.
- Prepare desserts with fruits and whole grains, such as apple crisp.
- Sprinkle wheat germ into your cereals or smoothies.
- Use whole-grain tortillas or pita breads to make healthy chips for dips or salsas.
- Use whole-grain pasta, whole-grain bread for sandwiches, and even whole-grain pizza bread.

FACT

Whole oats are a rich source of soluble fiber. Studies show that consuming 10–25 grams of soluble fiber per day can lower cholesterol by 10 percent. Portions that contain as little as 5–10 grams of soluble fiber can lower LDL cholesterol by as much as 5 percent. Three-quarters of a cup of uncooked oatmeal or ½ cup of oat bran contains 3 grams of soluble fiber.

Increasing Good Fats—Vegetable Oils, Nuts, and Fish

Research shows that the types of fats you eat strongly affect your cholesterol levels. While saturated and trans fats increase your LDL or bad cholesterol, unsaturated fats (including monounsaturated fats and polyunsaturated fats) actually reduce levels of bad cholesterol and increase levels of good cholesterol. Unsaturated fats are found in plant-based products such as most vegetable oils, nuts, seeds, and whole grains. The one nonplant source of these good fats is deepwater or fatty fish, which is a rich source of polyunsaturated fat.

Dietary fat is not the enemy. Heart-protective unsaturated fats play an important part in a healthy diet. The key is to try to watch what type of fat you eat—reduce saturated fats, eliminate trans fats, and then replace those fats with unsaturated fats in the diet. This does not give you permission to consume as much fat as you want as long as it is "healthy" fat. Remember, every gram of fat has over twice as many calories as a gram of protein. To maintain a healthy weight, you still want to eat only a small portion of healthy fats. Here are some tips on how to incorporate unsaturated fats into your daily diet:

- Cook with unsaturated liquid vegetable oils such as canola, safflower, grape seed, or, ideally, olive oil, which has shown to have the most benefits.
- If you must use some sort of butter or margarine, buy tub or liquid margarines with an unsaturated vegetable oil, such as soybean oil, as the first ingredient.
- Throw a few nuts or sesame seeds into your morning cereal. Foods that contain monounsaturated fats include almonds, cashews, peanuts, and walnuts.
- Spread natural peanut butter on celery sticks or green peppers for a healthy snack.
- Dip bread in limited amounts of olive oil instead of spreading on butter.
- Enjoy deepwater fish on occasion.
- Use flax seeds or powder as a topping or ingredient in grain dishes.

Omega-3 Fatty Acids

Another important heart-health benefit is found in polyunsaturated fats that include omega-3 (linolenic) and omega-6 (linoleic) fatty acids. Researchers have found that omega-3 fatty acids have an anti-inflammatory effect. They also reduce the likelihood of forming blood clots, help blood vessels relax or dilate, and can lower levels of LDL cholesterol. The primary source of omega-3 fatty acids is fish. Fish that come from cold, deep water are the best source of omega-3s. The American Heart Association recommends eating fatty fish at least twice a week. More recent information, however, about high mercury levels in fish and high carcinogen levels in farmed fish has caused concern, so be careful about the fish you buy.

Flaxseed and Flaxseed Oil

Flaxseed also contains high levels of omega-3 fatty acids and does not present the same mercury or carcinogenic concerns as fish. Using flaxseed, however, requires some care. Flaxseed must be ground up in order for the body to absorb the oils, and it cannot be cooked, as heat will destroy the oils in it.

ESSENTIAL

You can also take fish-oil supplements. A dose of about 4 grams of fish oil is considered beneficial. Finding high-quality supplements, however, is always a concern. Search for those from highly reputable producers that affirm the oils have been filtered for toxins such as mercury.

If you decide to add flaxseed into your diet, grind the seeds before you eat them. You can sprinkle ground flaxseed on cereal. Remember to store flaxseed in the refrigerator so the oil does not go rancid. If you purchase flaxseed oil, you can use it in salad dressings or on pasta, but do not cook with it. Based on results from research studies, the best amount to consume to achieve cholesterol-lowering results is 50 grams per day. Any amount is likely beneficial, though.

Raise a Glass to the Benefits of Moderate Drinking

Excessive drinking of alcohol is never a good practice. Heavy drinking can lead to high blood pressure and heart rhythm problems, as well as liver damage. For women, studies show that alcohol intake increases the risk of breast cancer. According to government statistics, up to 10 percent of U.S. adults misuse alcohol. Abstention from alcohol is the best practice for people who cannot enjoy it in moderation.

For those who can enjoy alcoholic beverages in moderation, however, studies show that alcohol consumption is associated with a lower risk of death from heart disease. Scientists have not identified the precise reasons why low amounts of alcohol consumption may reduce the risk of heart disease. Some experts theorize that it may be because it increases HDL cholesterol. Furthermore, the benefits occur regardless of which alcoholic beverage is consumed, meaning it is simply the ethanol in the alcohol that provides the positive results. Though low amounts of alcohol reduce cardiovascular risk, alcohol can increase the risk for many other diseases. Alcohol consumption comes with an increased risk of liver disease, gastritis, pancreatic disease, cancer, and many more diseases. These risks certainly outweigh any benefits in those who drink a significant amount of alcohol.

FACT

One drink is equal to 5 ounces of wine, 12 ounces of beer, or 1½ ounces of eighty-proof whiskey. For heart-health benefits, consume drinks with meals. No one should begin drinking alcoholic beverages if they do not already drink alcohol.

For wine enthusiasts, the news is even better. In addition to the HDL-raising benefits of alcohol, red wine also contains phytochemicals. These are plant-based chemicals that provide health benefits when consumed. The grape skins used in making red wine are full of compounds known as flavonoids. Flavonoids are known to help prevent LDL cholesterol from oxidizing and turning into the kind of early plaque that may adhere to arterial walls. Flavonoids also prevent blood clots, further reducing risk of a heart attack or stroke.

Regardless of any cardiovascular benefit, no one should ever increase alcohol consumption to, in theory, improve his health. While it may provide some cardiovascular benefit, this benefit comes with other risks. Generally, those who drink socially may have their cardiovascular profile improved somewhat, while anyone who drinks as often as daily should consider cutting down.

How to Read Food Labels

Eating right can help you feel better, give you more energy, manage your weight more effectively, and help you live a longer life with less risk of disability and disease. You know that you want to decrease the saturated fats, trans fats, and simple sugars in your diet and increase the monounsaturated and polyunsaturated fats, whole foods, and complex carbohydrates. But where do you begin? First, you need to understand how to read food labels. Next, you need some tips for navigating the aisles of your favorite grocery store.

What to Look For

The U.S. Food and Drug Administration regulates food labels. Labels must include not only a list of nutrients but also a list of ingredients. These are both sources of valuable information. In the nutrient list, the important items to check include the total fats and the breakdown of the types of fats included as well as the total carbohydrates and breakdown of fiber and sugar.

Aim for approximately 300–350 grams of complex carbohydrates, of which at least 20–30 grams are fiber. Also aim for at least 60 grams of lean protein daily, though you may need more if younger or an athlete. With fat, try to limit consumption to a maximum of 60 grams daily, but aim for less. Make sure to maximize unsaturated fat and minimize saturated and trans fat.

In the total fat section, check to see how much saturated fat and total fat are listed. Remember, "bad" fats that you should limit or avoid are saturated fat, trans fat, and cholesterol. "Good" fats that you can include are monounsaturated and polyunsaturated fats.

In the carbohydrate section of the label, check how much dietary fiber and sugar is in the product. Select foods that are higher in dietary fiber and as low as possible in sugar. When making a buying decision, compare products to find those that contain good fats instead of bad fats and that are high in fiber and whole grains.

Understanding the List of Ingredients

The ingredient list also provides a wealth of valuable information. Ingredients are listed in order of magnitude, with the items used in larger amounts listed first and smallest amounts at the end. Try to choose foods that feature grains, lean proteins, and fruits and vegetables at the start of the list, and have the fat and oil ingredients toward the end of the list.

Choose products that list the specific type of vegetable oil—olive oil, for example—rather than labels that use a generic "vegetable oil" listing. Often when manufacturers use the term vegetable oil, the product includes tropical oils such as palm or coconut that contain saturated fats, rather than the healthier monounsaturated and polyunsaturated fats. To avoid trans fats, stay away from products that list hydrogenated or partially hydrogenated vegetable oils.

When it comes to grain products, choose products with the words "whole," "whole wheat," or "whole grain" in front of the grain ingredient, as well as terms like "bran" or "germ." Sometimes food manufacturers will use enriched flour and dye it a brown color to make it appear like a whole grain. If the ingredient list shows enriched flour as the main ingredient, the grains are highly processed, even if it is enriched "wheat" flour. These are not whole grains, and the product is likely to be high in sugar and low in fiber. Read carefully.

Take Your Time

Be prepared to spend a little more time on your grocery shopping to allow yourself time to read labels. However, once you have selected foods you like that prominently feature healthful ingredients, you can return to your faster style of moving through aisles and throwing items in your shopping basket.

As you work your way through the fine print on labels, keep in mind that you are what you eat. This task of careful shopping, while tedious and time consuming at first, will pay great dividends to your better health in the long run and ultimately will become fairly quick and easy.

Your Shopping List

An important strategy that can go a long way toward improving your food choices is to prepare a shopping list before you go to the store. This helps you resist the newest, flashiest, and trendiest food products that are designed to catch your eye.

Note that the outer edges of the store tend to have the healthiest foods. These include the fresh fruits and vegetables, meats, breads, and dairy products. The inner aisles are filled with processed foods and ready-to-eat preparations that are full of saturated and trans fats, sugar, and salt. Remember that you want to select a balance of foods from each of the food groups.

From the bread and cereal group, choose whole-grain products like breads and muffins. You can also buy whole-grain pita bread, tortillas, pasta, and rice cakes. Choose whole-grain flour for baking and items such as brown or wild rice and whole corn or flour tortillas. Select whole-grain, unsweetened cereals or whole-grain hot cereals like oatmeal.

ESSENTIAL

As a careful shopper, over time you may become familiar with the manufacturers that create the healthier foods you want. You can gravitate toward those brands with more assurance that you are selecting items that will both taste good and be good for you. When purchasing something for the first time, it is still a good idea to check out the ingredients, no matter who the manufacturer.

From the fruit and vegetable group, select a variety of fresh foods. Today's frozen and canned vegetables can have as much nutritional value as fresh vegetables. If you're busy, you may have concerns that stocking up on fresh fruits and vegetables is wasteful. Go ahead and buy frozen products. If you buy canned vegetables, either go with a low-sodium variety or rinse the vegetables before serving. Canned fruits should come packed in juice, not syrup.

Another time saver is packaged, prewashed, presliced vegetables. These are ideal for snacks and salads. They may cost slightly more, but if they help you incorporate more vegetables into your diet, you will save more in the long run from your health dividends as you age. Fruit and vegetable juices are also good selections, especially if you can find fresh juices. Also be sure the fruit juice you buy is either 100 percent fruit juice or juice and water with no added sugar.

When choosing dairy and meat, remember the guidelines you learned earlier in this chapter. Look for low-fat or nonfat milk, cheese, and yogurt and lean cuts of meat. You can also select alternative sources of protein such as beans, nuts, and lentils.

Meal Planning for Health

Maintaining healthy nutrition does require some planning. However, with a minimal amount of organization, you can keep health-enhancing foods in your refrigerator and cupboards. Incorporate even a handful of these suggestions into your daily life and, before you realize it, you will have shifted to a healthier overall eating pattern. Each of these changes becomes easier with time and eventually can become automatic.

QUESTION

Which types of cooking oils should I buy?
Choose either monounsaturated vegetable oils, which include olive, canola, peanut, avocado, almond, hazelnut, and pecan, or polyunsaturated vegetable oils, such as corn, safflower, sunflower, sesame, soybean, and cottonseed.

Breakfast

Breakfast is the most important meal of the day because it ends the long period of body starvation, otherwise known as sleep. That is how breakfast earned its name: you are breaking the fast. It's also a wonderful opportunity to eat fiber-rich foods. Plan to include a combination of fiber-rich and protein-rich foods, along with either a fruit or vegetable serving. Great sources of fiber for breakfast include hot or cold whole grain cereals and breads. Breakfast protein can come from nonfat or low-fat dairy products such as milk. You can add fruits or vegetables either by drinking one glass of juice or by mixing fruit with your cereal or having it on the side. Another great breakfast option is a smoothie. These are easy to make in a blender with or without low-fat milk, some fruits, and wheat germ or ground flaxseed. All of these options can help you start your day on the right foot.

Lunch

Lunch is another great opportunity for a rich source of fiber and more fruits and vegetables. Try sandwiches on hearty whole-grain breads with fresh tomatoes, lettuce, and sprouts. You can also try using whole-grain pitas, tortillas, or wraps. You may prefer whole-grain pasta. For vegetable sources of protein, use bean dips such as hummus on a sandwich or nuts on the side.

FACT

Simple sugars are not "bad" in and of themselves, but when consumed in excess can have a harmful effect on cholesterol levels. Studies show that a diet high in simple sugars, which includes refined carbohydrates (enriched-flour breads and pastas) and hard candy, actually increases triglyceride levels and decreases levels of HDL or good cholesterol, in addition to promoting insulin resistance, an early form of type 2 diabetes.

If packing a lunch, include a vegetable and some fruit. For example, take some prewashed, prepackaged baby carrots or celery sticks. Or slice up a bell pepper into sticks. Easily portable fruits include apples, bananas, oranges, nectarines, grapes, and pears. There are also numerous types of prepackaged sliced fruits for your convenience. Try to eat fruits that are fresh and in season.

Salads are a great lunch that can be made more filling by adding beans or starches such as whole-grain pastas. Soups are a fantastic source of multiple vegetables and beans, but watch your salt intake, as that can raise blood pressure. If you combine soups or salads with some hearty whole-grain breads or muffins, you can have a satisfying and nutrient-packed meal. For dessert, try some fresh fruit or poached, baked, or frozen fruits, such as poached pears, baked apples, or fresh fruit sorbets.

Dinner

For dinner, try to shift the emphasis to a vegetable- and grain-based main course with any meat dishes on the side. Or, in meals that call for sauces, use a combination of vegetables and meats to reduce the total amount of meat that you consume. For example, you can cut the amount of meat in stew in half and instead add in extra carrots, celery, and mushrooms. You can try chili with beans and no meat, or use ground turkey instead of beef and add more vegetables instead of meats. Try enjoying stir-fried vegetable dishes with only a small amount of skinless chicken, or simply use tofu instead of any meat product.

ALERT

It is not a good idea to transition immediately to a diet filled with massive amounts of fiber. Add more fiber-rich foods such as beans and whole grains gradually. This helps prevent constipation and too much gas, neither of which are pleasant experiences. Be sure to drink plenty of fluids and also to follow bean preparation instructions carefully.

Keep in mind that when you eat beans, peas, or lentils together with a dairy product or grains such as bread or rice, you can obtain the same amount of protein from your meal as if you had consumed a meat dish. Other benefits of eating more beans instead of meat is that they are much more affordable, they contain no saturated fats and no cholesterol, they are nutrient dense, and they are valuable sources of dietary fiber.

If you use canned beans in your foods, try to buy low-sodium varieties and use the liquid that they come packed in for cooking. That liquid is rich in soluble fiber—that's why it has that thick consistency.

Heart-Healthy Dining for Winning Results

Dietary changes are very powerful. Blood-cholesterol levels show signs of improvement in as few as three to four weeks. Over several months, LDL levels can be reduced through dietary changes by as much as 60 percent! This reduces the risk of suffering a debilitating or deadly heart attack or stroke.

Keep in mind, however, that you must make a lifestyle change toward a healthier pattern of eating and not treat this as a short-term, fad diet for quick and easy weight loss. Eating healthy for life represents a commitment—to yourself and to those you love—to make a daily difference in supporting health through the foods that you eat. Treats are definitely a part of that picture, but for the most part, your daily diet will be one that is full of nutrient-dense, health-enhancing foods for a longer, healthier, and more enjoyable life.

CHAPTER 10

Successful Weight Management

Healthy weight management is an important part of a healthy lifestyle. Maintaining a healthy weight requires understanding what causes weight gain and the key strategies to prevent it, as you will learn in this chapter. A healthy weight requires a combination of good nutrition, consistent physical activity, and effective stress management, which are important factors of a healthy cholesterol profile as well. When you keep your weight at a healthy level, you will live longer with more energy and fewer disabilities.

What Is a Healthy Weight?

A healthy weight is one that minimizes your risk of illness and disease and falls within the range of weight appropriate for your height. A person may suffer from poor health if overly heavy. Similarly, a person can experience poor health if overly thin. Therefore, a reasonable weight goal is in between those two extremes. This can fall within a broad range, as people come in a variety of sizes and shapes due to strong genetic factors. Each person should find his own healthy weight for his own body type.

Understanding Body Composition

It's not just the size of the package that is important; it's what is inside the package that counts. Your body is composed of fat mass and lean body mass. Together, this is referred to as your body composition. Ideally, you want to keep the percentage of fat quite a bit lower than the percentage of nonfat mass. (Your nonfat mass includes your bones, organs, and muscle.) And, if you decide to lose weight, you want to lose fat, not valuable muscle tissue that gives you strength and support.

FACT

The good news for those who are overweight is that even a small reduction in weight, as little as 10 percent of total body weight, leads to remarkable improvements in health. For example, research subjects who lost 10 percent of total body weight have experienced reductions in high blood pressure, blood glucose, bad cholesterol levels, and disease as well as improvements in body composition.

Just because a person appears to be thin does not make him healthy. Some people who are thin in appearance are actually unhealthy when it comes to body composition. Typically, they are weak, sedentary, and may be smokers. They may eat very little food and have an unbalanced diet. Oftentimes, people with this type of profile believe they are healthy as long as they are thin. They could not be more mistaken.

Being significantly underweight poses serious threats to good health. For premenopausal women, being too underweight can lead to infertility or osteoporosis. People who suffer from disorders such as anorexia or bulimia also experience poor health. In particular, people who are anorectic will consume muscle tissue from their body's stores to survive when fat stores are depleted, including tissue from the heart muscle.

At the same time, a person who may be more stocky and robust in appearance but who exercises regularly, eats a balanced diet of nutrient-rich fresh foods, and who does not smoke is much healthier.

The message, therefore, is not that thin is in or that every person must have the same body. Rather, you should aim to maintain a weight that is healthy for you and your body type.

All Body Fat Is Not Equal

To make matters even more complex, researchers have found that the amount of body fat is not the only factor that is important. What is equally (if not more) significant is where the fat is deposited on your body. Studies show that people whose bodies store fat around the abdominal area, also referred to as an apple-shaped body, are at higher risk of heart disease, stroke, high blood pressure, and type 2 diabetes than those who are more pear shaped and carry their excess fat around their legs and thighs. Unfortunately, it's hard to dictate where your fat goes, but you can dictate how much of it you have.

QUESTION

Why does abdominal fat create a higher risk of heart disease than fat elsewhere?
The exact reasons why abdominal fat poses greater risks are not known, but one factor that may contribute is the fact that abdominal fat puts greater stress on internal organs that become surrounded with fat.

To determine whether you have abdominal obesity, you need to measure your waist circumference. For purposes of this measurement, your waist is considered to be halfway between the lowest rib and the top of your hipbone, measured when you are upright and your trunk is perpendicular to the floor. A waist circumference of greater than forty inches for men, or greater than thirty-five inches for women, may indicate a higher risk of heart disease. Abdominal obesity is also considered one of the risk factors of the metabolic syndrome.

The Body Mass Index

Another method to assess whether your weight may put you at risk is to calculate your body mass index (BMI). The BMI expresses weight relative to height. It provides a general guideline to check whether you are in a healthy weight range. A high BMI score may indicate increased risks for heart disease, high blood pressure, type 2 diabetes, and high cholesterol. BMI guidelines are not accurate for estimating risks for people who are healthy at higher weight levels, such as muscular competitive athletes or pregnant women. These guidelines also do not apply to growing children or frail and sedentary older adults.

Instructions for calculating your BMI are included in Appendix B. If your BMI is greater than 25, you fall into the category of overweight. A BMI between 18.5 and 24.9 is considered a healthy weight. If your BMI score is less than 18.5, you are considered to be underweight.

Beyond Your Looks

Losing excess fat is not only an important factor in reducing the risk of cardiovascular disease but also in reducing the risk of many diseases, including gallbladder disease, type 2 diabetes, and cancer.

In addition to the reduced risk for numerous diseases, losing weight provides multiple physical, mental, and emotional benefits. People who lose excess weight feel better, have more energy, have fewer aches and pains, and can enjoy a higher quality of life. People may also experience an improved sense of self-esteem and a feeling of greater control over their lives that leads to a greater sense of self-confidence.

Excess weight strains your heart and your circulatory system. Your heart must work harder to pump more blood through your body, causing higher blood pressure. Extra weight also strains your musculoskeletal system and puts greater stress on your joints, increasing arthritis and back pain.

People who carry excess weight are more likely to have certain risk factors for cardiovascular disease, including high LDL cholesterol, low HDL cholesterol, high triglycerides, type 2 diabetes, or high blood pressure. At the same time, when people who are overweight lose excess body fat, even as few as five to ten pounds, they can typically expect reductions in their total cholesterol, LDL, and triglycerides, accompanied by increases in HDL. All of these benefits combined are much greater than the sum of their parts.

Causes of Weight Gain

In simplistic terms, one can say that the cause of weight gain is taking in excess calories. But this does not take into full consideration the complex social factors that make it difficult to live an active lifestyle, to enjoy wholesome fresh foods, and to separate emotional factors from the need to eat. Furthermore, as researchers learn more and more about the differences among people's metabolic profiles, it seems that depending on what types of foods are consumed, some people are more prone to gain weight easily and to have a more difficult time losing it. The overall picture is complex, but a few simple factors play key roles.

Supersizing of Foods

In this day and age, it is easy for people to overeat. The supersizing of food portions by food manufacturers adds to this tendency. Since most of the cost of food production is in the labor and not in the raw materials, food producers have financial incentives to increase the size of food products in order to attract more customers. The increased amount of cost involved in providing a larger serving size is outweighed by the greater number of customers who purchase their product, since it is perceived as a better value or more food for the money. This perception of value by consumers, however, fails to take into consideration that they are actually purchasing more food than they need. And all that excess consumption leads to excess weight. Consumers might think they are paying just a little bit more for a lot more food, but in actuality they are paying much more for the harm the extra food does to their bodies.

In fact, this issue is so prevalent that the U.S. Federal Trade Commission, and more recently the U.S. Food and Drug Administration, recommends manufacturers re-examine the portion sizes on food labels. The FTC and FDA have made this recommendation based on the fact that "they [food labels] may significantly understate the amount of particular foods and calories that people typically consume."

Officials at the FTC believe that current food-labeling practices confuse consumers over serving sizes so that consumers "may underestimate the number of calories and other nutrients that they eat." For example, a typical three-ounce bag of chips is labeled as "two servings" but packaged as a single serving. Twenty-ounce soft drinks are also packaged as a single serving but described as two servings on the food label. The FTC recommends that the FDA look at whether serving-size listings are "sufficiently clear and prominent."

Until government officials clear up current labeling practices, however, it is up to you to make judgments about serving sizes on your own. Generally, serving sizes are much smaller than typical portion sizes, so you consume more fat, carbohydrates, and calories than are listed for a single serving. To get a better idea of how much you consume, you must try to determine the number of servings you are eating by paying attention to the serving size as compared to your portion size. Take time to read food labels carefully, and compare the weight of the package with what is noted as the weight of a serving on the label. Also, read the serving-size guidelines at the end of this chapter carefully.

Emotional Overeating

While emotional overeating may not rise to the level of a clinical eating disorder, many people overeat in response to cues that are completely unrelated to hunger. Stress can play a role, as can environmental factors in the home. For example, if your parents rewarded you with a food treat when you accomplished tasks, you may continue to give yourself this type of treat when you finish something as an adult. Similarly, if food was used to cope with emotions rather than discussing, facing, or experiencing them, it can continue to play that role in adult life.

Keeping a journal can be helpful for people who find that they eat in response to these types of emotional cues rather than to true feelings of hunger. In the journal, you can record what triggered an eating episode, what you were thinking and feeling at the time, and what feelings you were avoiding by eating. This process may be very revealing as you start to unravel some of your more unconscious eating behaviors that lead to over-consumption of food.

ESSENTIAL

Researchers suggest that if you eat the foods you really like in measured amounts with meals and avoid them when you are hungry, you can reduce your cravings. The reason is that by giving in to your body's desire for certain foods, you can train your body to want that treat even more. For example, if you only eat chocolate when you're ravenous, you can increase the strength of your cravings.

Eating Highly Refined, Processed Foods

Another factor that can contribute to overeating is choosing foods that are highly refined and processed. In this case, the overeating often occurs in response to genuine hunger cues. For example, breads and pastas that are made with enriched flour rather than with whole grains lack fiber that provides important feelings of fullness and satiety. Drinking juices instead of eating fruits is also another missed opportunity to eat fiber-rich foods.

Fiber, both soluble and insoluble, is critically important to health. Not only does it provide roughage that is good for digestion, but it also lowers cholesterol levels and makes you feel full. It truly is hard to overeat when your meals are filled with wholesome fresh fruits, vegetables, and whole grains that have bulk and are steadily absorbed.

Lack of Physical Activity

Living an active lifestyle in today's technology-driven world is a challenge. It is actually much easier to live a sedentary life today than it is to live an active life. Without a conscious effort to move, it's actually quite easy to remain inactive all day long. When this lack of movement is combined with overconsumption of foods, it's easy to see how the combination can quickly add to increased weight gain.

Loss of Lean Body Mass

An aspect of the picture that affects metabolism and activity levels is the natural decline in lean body mass that occurs with aging. After the age of thirty-five, both men and women lose approximately one-third to one-half pound of muscle each year. If your total weight is not changing, this means that this loss of lean body mass has been replaced by an equivalent gain of fat mass. Although your weight may not have changed, the difference between these two types of tissues is extremely significant from the standpoint of weight management.

The loss of lean body mass means your body is composed of less of the metabolically more active tissue as well as a decrease in the muscle that provides strength to move and accomplish physical tasks. So not only is the body burning fewer calories even at rest, but it also becomes more tired and less capable of doing things such as walking up the stairs, running after children, and lifting and carrying grocery bags.

ESSENTIAL

Health benefits can be gained from even a modest weight loss. You do not need to become a size two or look like a cover model. You just need to be sure that you lose the weight in a healthy way. As with cholesterol, blood pressure, blood sugar, and smoking, even small changes in your weight can go a long way.

This is the beginning of a cycle of reduced daily physical activity that leads to even more fat gain. Over time, the ratio of fat becomes high and the amount of lean low. The older adult may no longer have the strength even to climb a flight of stairs or get up and move around at all, and the pounds can easily add up. Basically, the less you move, the less muscle you have and more weight you gain, so the less you want to move. The key is to interrupt and turn around this vicious cycle. The more you move, the slimmer you will be and the more muscle and energy you'll have, motivating you to keep moving.

Why Dieting Does Not Work

Diets that involve simply avoiding food altogether, known as starvation diets, don't work. You need to eat nutritious foods to lose weight and keep it down. When you starve yourself, you lose both fat and hard-earned muscle tissue. This loss of lean body mass from dieting results in a decreased resting metabolic rate, similar to when people lose lean body mass as they age. Therefore, just starving yourself will slow your metabolism down, yet you will eventually eat more due to your hunger, with a slower metabolism to burn less of what you eat. This is called yo-yo dieting—the tendency to lose and regain the same weight over and over again, rather than making any permanent changes in weight management. Some researchers believe this is even more detrimental to health than not dieting at all.

ALERT

If you're out of shape, a new regular exercise program can build up your muscles. It may seem discouraging at first because you may see a weight gain. (Remember, muscle weighs more than fat.) But for every pound of muscle you gain, you also burn about thirty to fifty more calories a day, for the same amount of effort. Over time, the added muscle will help you lose and manage your weight.

Healthy weight loss should occur at the rate of no more than one to two pounds per week. At this healthy rate, you are losing body fat rather than muscle tissue. You are also more likely to keep it off and avoid the yo-yo syndrome.

What Does Work

The bottom line when it comes to weight management is that lifestyle changes will help bring your weight to a healthy level. Depending on how much excess fat you have, this process may take a longer time. However, any lifestyle changes you are able to make will improve your health and feelings of well-being.

Do Your Best to Be Your Best

Managing your weight is part of a healthy lifestyle. To achieve success, it's best to make changes gradually and to have realistic expectations. The following tips can help you get started:

- Examine your eating habits. Are you meeting the necessary requirements?
- Portion size matters. Learn what healthy single servings of food are, and adjust your portion sizes.
- Get active each and every day. Every movement counts.
- Incorporate strength or weight training to increase your lean body mass.

As you improve your daily habits, instead of focusing on changes in your scale weight, notice changes in how you feel. Do you have more energy? Are you feeling stronger? Are you sleeping better at night?

If you're the type who needs a goal in the form of a number, such as weight, to keep you motivated, think about measuring your progress in other ways. Get your cholesterol and blood sugar levels tested. Check whether your resting heart rate and blood pressure levels are going down. Most important, know you're doing the best you can for your long-term well-being.

ESSENTIAL

The best approach for weight management is one that is grounded in the following basics: healthy nutrition, regular physical activity that includes lifestyle activity, and stress management.

Avoid Overeating

While it is important to eat a diet full of foods that enhance health and to avoid eating those foods that can be harmful to health, keep in mind that overeating any foods can lead to excess weight that is harmful to health. One of the ways to avoid overeating is to learn what a reasonable serving size should look like. Here are some helpful visual cues:

- One serving of fresh fruit or vegetables is about the size of a tennis ball.
- One serving of canned fruit or cooked vegetables is about the size of a computer mouse.
- One serving of dried fruit is about the size of a golf ball.
- One serving of fruit as juice measures ¾ cup.*
- One serving of vegetable juice measures 1 cup.*
- One serving of sliced bread is about the size of a centimeter.
- One serving of cold cereal is about the size of a baseball.
- One serving of hot cereal is about the size of an English muffin.
- One serving of rice or pasta is about the size of a regular scoop of ice cream.

*It is recommended that as many of your servings as possible come from whole fruit and vegetables, with no more than half of your fruit and vegetable servings from fruit juice, since juice does not provide the same amount of dietary fiber as the fruit itself.

Restaurants tend to promote overeating with large portions, and most do not list their ingredients or nutritional information, leaving you ignorant of their contents. There are several strategies you can use to avoid overeating when you are eating out: share a main course with a friend; order a meal of various side dishes; or simply take half of the order home to eat later. Also, more and more restaurants have a healthier menu, typically meals with more vegetables and grilled lean meats as opposed to fried foods. If you have the opportunity to plan ahead, restaurants will often list the nutritional information for their menu on their website. Occasionally, you can get a copy of the menu's nutritional information on request.

Keep in mind that lifestyle habits are not easy to change. Be gentle with yourself and appreciate your small successes on a daily basis. Over time, you will find that your life has transformed in so many more ways than simply managing your weight. The weight that you lose, whatever the amount, represents your body's quest to find its best balance in the midst of a lifestyle dedicated to creating health.

CHAPTER 11

Getting Active

Along with eating a balanced diet, being active on most days of the week is critical to creating health. Getting active for health does not mean spending hours at the gym. In fact, you never even have to go to the gym to get the amount of exercise proved to improve your health, though a gym can often help. This chapter will explain why physical activity is beneficial and how you can get moving to enjoy those results.

Physical Activity Benefits Heart Health

People are designed to be active creatures. Not so long ago, people had to perform physical work to feed, clothe, and shelter themselves. Modern living has changed all of that, but it cannot change the fundamental need of people to move and use their bodies in order to maintain optimum functioning. As average levels of physical activity have declined, medical professionals have observed an accompanying decline in the body's physical functioning. Researchers are also studying the relationship of physical inactivity with decline in mental functioning.

Numerous studies now substantiate the fact that a minimal amount of physical movement is not only beneficial but essential. Many aspects of aging, such as the loss of strength, balance, and the ability to move and care for oneself, were formerly viewed as a natural result of the aging process. Research today shows that many of these consequences are not actually the result of aging. Rather, they are the result of disuse of the body and a failure to take advantage of its physical capabilities. To retain your vitality and energy, you need to keep yourself physically active.

How Does Activity Affect the Heart?

Physical inactivity is a major risk factor for heart disease. The heart is a muscle that benefits from regular use to keep it and the circulatory system healthy. When a person is inactive, the heart muscle is weaker. With each beat, an unfit heart muscle pumps a lower volume of blood than a stronger, fit heart.

Because less blood is pumped, the heart has to beat more frequently to ensure adequate circulation of blood around the body. This more rapid heart rate can also result in an increase in blood pressure over time, causing stiffness and hardening of the arteries and affecting the health of the circulatory system. In contrast, when the heart is strong and healthy, stroke volume is strong. The heart rate is slower, and a more healthy tone is maintained in the arterial walls.

Increasing physical activity has many heart disease benefits. It decreases your blood pressure and your resistance to insulin, thereby decreasing the chance of developing diabetes. It also leads to an increase in the levels of HDL, or good cholesterol. This change is independent of any weight loss that may also occur as increased activity burns up more calories. Physical activity also lowers LDL and triglyceride levels.

Studies show that regular physical activity not only lowers bad cholesterol and triglycerides and increases good cholesterol, but that it also reduces risk of death from all causes, reduces feelings of depression and anxiety, and helps build and maintain healthy bones, muscles, and joints.

FACT

Only moderate amounts of physical activity are required to reverse the downward spiral toward ill health. A moderate amount of activity can mean as little as thirty minutes of brisk walking on most days of the week.

Studies also show that people who are physically active after a first heart attack have a significantly lower risk of having a second heart attack when compared with people who remained inactive.

How Much Activity Is Necessary?

According to guidelines issued by the U.S. Surgeon General, the U.S. Department of Health and Human Services, and the National Heart, Lung, and Blood Institute, the minimum amount of activity for health includes the following factors:

- Should continue for at least 30 minutes total
- Can be accumulated in bouts as short as 8–10 minutes
- Should be of moderate intensity, such as brisk walking
- Should occur on most, preferably all, days of the week
- Should include some resistance exercise and stretching during the week

The guidelines also note that more activity and a higher intensity will provide greater health and fitness benefits. The general guidelines listed above set forth minimum amounts of activity necessary to enjoy health benefits.

ALERT

According to surveys, only 40 percent of adults meet the minimum activity recommendation to provide health benefits of thirty minutes on most days of the week.

What Is Moderate Activity?

Research shows that activity can come in a variety of ways and still provide health benefits. The good news is that with so many activities to choose from, you are likely to find something that you enjoy and are able to incorporate into your life on a regular basis. The following are examples of moderate amounts of physical activity:

▼ **EXAMPLES OF MODERATE AMOUNTS OF ACTIVITIES**

Types of Activity	Length of Time
Playing volleyball	45 minutes
Playing touch football	30–45 minutes
Walking 1¾ miles	35 minutes (20-minute mile, or pace of 3 miles/hour)
Basketball (shooting baskets)	30 minutes
Bicycling 5 miles	30 minutes
Walking 2 miles	30 minutes (15-minute mile, or pace of 4 miles/hour)
Water aerobics	30 minutes
Swimming laps	20 minutes
Wheelchair basketball	20 minutes

You can also perform some activities that are performed at a higher intensity, such as bicycling, jumping rope, running, shoveling snow, or climbing stairs for a shorter amount of time (fifteen minutes or so) to get similar results. However, it is not necessary to do high-intensity exercises to achieve health benefits; moderate-intensity exercise can improve heart health. The most important thing is to get moving!

The key to maintaining an exercise regimen is to find something that you can and will do regularly, and that you do it for at least thirty minutes on most days of the week. Remember that you can break up those thirty minutes. For example, you can take a ten-minute morning walk, run a quick errand on a bicycle at noon for ten minutes, and then take another ten-minute walk at the end of the day.

Lifestyle Activity Is Important

Many people are so conditioned to thinking that exercise means going to the gym that they forget that everyday life presents them with numerous opportunities to get active during the day. If you have time to go to the gym, that's fantastic. But if you don't, do not despair. You can create movement opportunities during your day that make a difference. Look for every opportunity for activity. Make a schedule. Give up TV time. Do whatever it takes to find time for activity.

ESSENTIAL

Keep in mind that studies show people who live an otherwise sedentary life and work out for one hour per day are not burning as many calories as people who do not go to the gym but who take part in lifestyle activities throughout the day. Constantly look for more activity opportunities in your life, whether more walking breaks, sports activities, or activities around the home.

Here are some examples of lifestyle activity:

- Walk to run an errand in the neighborhood, rather than taking a car.
- Play outdoor games with children instead of watching television together.
- Park farther away from the shop.
- Get off the train or bus one stop early and walk the rest of the way.
- Carry your groceries to your car or load them into your car yourself.
- Wash your car instead of taking it to the car wash.
- Rake leaves instead of using a leaf blower.
- Get up to switch appliances on or off instead of always using remote controls.
- Ride a bicycle for transportation instead of driving a car.

- Do some vigorous housecleaning such as vacuuming, sweeping, or mopping.

Be creative—find more and more ways you can move during your day. These activities all add up and make a difference. According to estimates for a 150-pound person, standing up for three ten-minute phone calls will burn twenty calories. In contrast, sitting for thirty minutes during those three phone calls burns only four calories. While sixteen calories may not seem like much, when it is repeated hour after hour, day after day, it and other small actions start to mean the difference between unwanted pounds and maintaining your ideal weight.

After you eat during the day, your blood is filled with sugars and fats, blood glucose and triglycerides, sources of fuel that you can use immediately. However, if you do not use up this energy, it ultimately ends up stored as fat. One of the keys to keeping all systems healthy is to use up this fuel for its intended purpose and stimulate your heart, lungs, muscles, and skeletal and nervous systems.

Exercise Your Way to a Healthy Heart

One of the best forms of exercise that provides a healthful challenge for the human body is walking. It is economical, easy to fit into your day, bears a low risk of injury, and is effective in improving health. Numerous studies show that people who walk regularly have less risk of death or disability from disease.

In addition to reducing the risks of heart disease, walking helps you enjoy many other benefits, including maintaining a healthy weight, improving the condition of bones and muscles, and reducing stress and tension.

FACT

A study showed that older men who started walking about two miles a day had a 50 percent lower risk of heart attack than men who walked only a quarter mile. In addition, the study found that the risk of a heart attack dropped an additional 15 percent for every additional half mile walked per day.

Your Exercise Program: The First Steps

You're ready to get going with your daily exercise, but you're not quite sure how to begin. That's natural. A regular exercise program does include a few details that you need to address. The following information provides you with everything you need to know to get moving.

Check with Your Health Care Provider

Before you get started with any exercise program, it is a good idea to check with your health care provider. If you are apparently healthy and under the age of sixty-five, then a moderate exercise program is probably fine. If, however, you are older or have any known chronic conditions such as arthritis, diabetes, or heart disease, you need to check with your health care provider. An exercise program is likely to have multiple benefits for you, but safe is always better than sorry. Check with your doctor in case there are any specific limitations you need to be aware of.

Find the Right Shoes

Your most important and significant investment is in the shoes you will wear. Take the time to find a comfortable, sturdy shoe that fits the needs of your foot and provides good arch support. Shoe technology these days is actually quite sophisticated. Go to a reputable athletic footwear store that allows returns if the shoe is not a good fit for you.

Consider eventually buying shoe inserts. Today's shoes do not come with insoles that last as long as the outer part of the shoe. Yet the cushioning that provides you with support is essential to keep you comfortable and prevent injury. When you purchase your shoes, ask the salesperson to also help you find an appropriate insole. This will make a tremendous difference in your long-term comfort.

Choose the Right Clothing and Accessories

As far as sportswear for exercise, you want to wear fabrics that breathe, such as cotton or polyester blends. Many modern fabrics also feature wicking qualities that draw your perspiration away from your skin. Women who need the extra support should wear an athletic sports bra.

Sun protection is also important—be sure to wear sunscreen. A hat is also a good idea to protect your face. Depending on how sensitive you are to sun exposure, you may want to purchase a hat that also shields the back of your neck. Sunglasses provide coverage for your eyes; choose a pair that is lightweight and comfortable. More than anything, you want your walks as enjoyable as possible.

FACT

Consider wearing bright colors for walking or running. Not only will they cheer you up, they will also help make sure that you are visible to any traffic. You can purchase reflector vests as well.

Stay Hydrated

Staying properly hydrated is essential for good health. If you are exercising for longer than an hour and are not near a water fountain, bringing your own water supply is a good idea. Some companies market fanny packs that serve as water bottle carriers that are handy for longer walks. Most important, remember to drink plenty of fluids before, during, and after your exercise. For moderate levels of exercise, plan on about five to seven ounces of water every fifteen to twenty minutes.

Consider a Pedometer

It is not necessary to purchase a pedometer, but it is a great tool to measure your progress and keep you motivated. You should take at least 10,000 steps a day, the equivalent of about five miles, but more is always better. The steps the pedometer measures do not require a particular intensity level or a specific duration. What they represent is that you have maintained a level of daily activity that contributes to your health.

The motivational aspect of the pedometer is that it helps you realize exactly how much you move around during the day. You can constantly try to increase the number of steps you take daily. This can help you become a more active person on a daily basis, which can make a significant difference in your overall caloric expenditure as well as your health and well-being.

CHAPTER 12

Stress Management for a Healthy Heart

Stress. Even the sound of the word evokes feelings of tension. Stress is a daily aspect of modern living. Stress can keep you motivated and even save your life. If unmanaged, however, stress can kill you. Excess stress weakens the immune system. Furthermore, stress can make any disease condition worse. In this chapter, you will discover what stress is, how stress contributes to heart disease, how you can identify stress, and what steps you can take to reduce stress and restore balance to your life.

What Is Stress?

Stress is actually a natural physiological response to something that triggers a feeling of fear or threat. This response, called fight or flight, is designed to help you survive life-threatening situations. The natural chemical response that affects your mind and body is like a miracle drug that can help save your life in the face of a dangerous emergency.

The Stress Response

The body's response to stress is stimulated by stress hormones like adrenaline and cortisol, released by your body to prepare you for action. Among other things, these stress hormones do the following:

- Increase your heart rate and blood pressure to pump an extra burst of oxygen-rich blood around your body so you can get moving
- Stop the flow of blood to your digestive system and skin by constricting arteries, saving blood flow for more needed areas
- Channel the increased blood flow to the brain and muscles by relaxing arteries
- Increase perspiration to cool the body
- Activate receptors that generate quick bursts of energy
- Speed up your breathing rate and open bronchial tubes to draw more oxygen-rich air into the lungs

When you look at all of these changes, it's easy to see how this chemically induced state of emergency preparedness is extremely useful in life-threatening situations.

ESSENTIAL

The stress response protects the body in a number of ways. It triggers the body to release blood sugar into the bloodstream to provide immediately available energy for fuel. It beefs up the blood-clotting mechanism in the event of potential injury. In addition, your body becomes extremely alert to enable you to immediately spot any signs of danger.

The modern challenge, however, is to manage the stress response, which can trigger when you're not in any physical danger. In fact, most contemporary stresses are mental and emotional. You find yourself stuck in traffic, missing deadlines at work. You worry about your family, your money, and your health. For some people, these stress levels stay high throughout the day. Both body and mind feel the strain, and the body gets no opportunity to physically release any of this tension energy.

How Stress Harms Health

Stress can harm health if it mounts to levels at which you feel you can no longer cope. This usually occurs after stress levels have remained high over a prolonged period of time.

The hormones like adrenaline and cortisol released during stressful situations raise blood sugar and constrict many of your blood vessels. This raises your blood pressure, increasing your cardiovascular risk. The increased blood sugar and hormones increase your LDL and triglycerides while decreasing your HDL. Like smoking, obesity, or lack of exercise, stress affects all aspects of your cardiovascular risk.

Other physical and mental symptoms of excessive stress include rapid pulse, chronic muscle tension, headaches, digestive problems, ulcers, infections, irritability, depression, anxiety, loss of ability to concentrate, altered sleeping or eating habits, and increased use of drugs or alcohol. Understanding stress and having skills to manage it effectively are important to your overall health and wellness.

Stress and Heart Disease

The American Heart Association does not include stress as one of the leading risk factors for heart disease. However, this may have more to do with the difficulty of separating stress from other risk factors, since stress contributes to various risk factors. In other words, it is difficult to prove that stress is an independent risk factor given that it also contributes to so many other risk factors, including smoking, physical inactivity, overeating, and high cholesterol, blood sugar, and blood pressure. The American Heart Association, however, does note that individual responses to stress may be a contributing factor to heart disease risk.

Stress and Heart Function

After studying the long-term effects of stress, some researchers believe that prolonged stress can cause damage to blood vessels. Stress hormones, to channel blood flow to essential areas in times of stress, will constrict. This constriction leads to endothelial dysfunction, a precursor to the development of atherosclerosis.

Over time, the blood vessels lose their ability to dilate effectively until the blood vessels cannot respond appropriately to changes in blood demands. For example, constricted arteries would fail to provide an increased blood flow to meet the needs of working muscles in the legs.

Identifying Stress in Your Life

Most contemporary stress-inducing situations are not dangerous in and of themselves. What makes them stressful is the way you react to them. Some people thrive in situations that make others miserably tense and anxious. For example, you may hate meeting deadlines, while a friend works productively under that type of pressure. If you are frequently rushed or competitive and feel overwhelmed by this, or you let small frustrations get to you, or you find it hard to forget your worries and relax, tackling your stress levels will most likely improve your health. At the same time, you can certainly make your life more enjoyable.

Other types of stress are not caused by your attitude, but are the product of a busy life. For example, if you are driving in heavy traffic and someone quickly cuts in front of you, that is a stressful situation. You have a legitimate fear for your safety, as a car accident could result. Your reaction, however, does not require you to burn off any physical energy. Rather, you remain seated in your car. You are likely to tighten your muscles and experience feelings of tension and anxiety as your body undergoes the physiological and biochemical changes associated with the fight-or-flight response.

Often, when you feel "stressed out," it is a generalized feeling of stress. If you take a moment to examine your situation, however, you will find that your feelings are actually the cumulative result of numerous individual pressures that have finally reached the boiling point. One of the first steps toward learning how to manage stress effectively is to identify these individual pressures.

ALERT

Numerous studies demonstrate that people who are more likely to become angry have about three times greater risk of having a heart attack or sudden cardiac death than those who are less prone to become angry. Other studies show that as people experience anger, they are more likely to have an arrhythmia or irregular heartbeat.

The next time you start to feel overwhelmed and stressed out, explore these feelings in greater depth. Ask yourself the following questions to determine what is causing these emotions:

- Am I overcommitted?
- Am I taking care of others and neglecting myself?
- Am I trying to accomplish everything on my own without asking for any support from anyone else?
- Are my expectations unrealistic?
- What is going on in my life right now that gives me a sense of struggle?
- Is what I stress over more important than my health and happiness?

If you are the type of person who finds it helpful to keep a journal, try to record things that trigger your stress. Write down what happened, what you were thinking or feeling, and how you reacted physically. This can give you valuable insight into the cumulative triggers you face throughout the day. Then consider the importance of those things and the importance of your long-term health and well-being. Consider the effects of stress on your health and mood and how that then affects those around you. Is what you stress over more concerning than premature death and disability? If not, then it is worth learning how to manage your stress.

When you start to identify the causes for your feelings and also note how you react to these stressors, you bring more awareness and understanding to your personal situation. Once you realize what triggers your stress, you are ready to consider taking realistic steps to cope with your personal matters.

Strategies for Dealing with Stress

It's important for your health and mental wellness that you feel a sense of control over your life. Making time to learn stress management skills and relaxation techniques can help you gain that control. Learning how to manage or eliminate some of the stressors in your life is also important for keeping your immune system strong, reducing your risk of illness, and improving your feelings of well-being.

Identify Priorities and Manage Time Effectively

Time management is a critical skill to develop to successfully manage stress. Everyone has the same number of hours in the day. Some people, however, are more effective managers of their time and priorities. To get organized, first identify your priorities. Next, make a realistic plan for how long it will take to get things done. Do the best you can, and remember to leave time for yourself.

If you feel that you need help in this area, consider taking a course in time or stress management. Consult your health care provider about available resources. You may want to enroll in a group course or work one on one with a counselor.

Rely on Social Support

Numerous studies have shown the positive affect of relationships on stress and health. Prioritizing and fostering those relationships is important not only for those around you, but for yourself as well. The more close ties you have with your family, friends, and community, the greater benefit to your health and happiness. Studies even indicate that pet ownership can contribute to heart health. Researchers have found that pet owners consistently have reduced stress reactions as measured by lower heart rates and blood pressures, especially when the pets are present.

Forgiveness is important to coping with difficult emotions. Negative feelings and stressful situations can adversely affect your health. When you forgive others for actions you feel were unfair or inappropriate, you can release or heal strong negative emotions.

Express Yourself Without Anger

Remember that people who get angry easily are much more likely to die from a heart attack. If you find that you are often irritated or annoyed, learn constructive methods to deal with disagreeable situations. Learn more effective communication skills to defuse conflicts. Make sure you are not allowing resentment to build up inside you. Over time, denial of anger can lead to unhealthy blowups or chronic negative feelings. The healthiest approach is to learn how to effectively express your feelings in positive and constructive ways.

It may help to remember some simple alternatives to becoming angry or frustrated in stressful situations. If possible, leave the scene of a stressful situation before it gets to you. Talk to someone you trust about how you feel or take some time on your own to brainstorm nonstressful ways to respond to a stressful issue. Most important, remember to breathe deeply and ask yourself, "In the scheme of things, does this really matter? Is this more important than my health and happiness?"

Make Time for Self-Care

One of the biggest contributors to feelings of stress is the sense that life is out of control. To avoid this, make time for yourself, just like taking time to exercise or eat healthy. You deserve time for your own self-care. For one thing, it supports your health, which in turn helps you better support those you care about. Take a moment to identify things that you enjoy, that bring you pleasure, and that are fun and restorative. Make it a point to incorporate these activities into your schedule.

It is never easy to change a habit. Unless stress is managed and the reasons for maintaining the behavioral change are foremost in your mind, old habits prevail. A calm, clear, and focused mind and a healthy, realistic attitude are important for achieving any goal. This holds equally true for the incorporation of healthy lifestyle habits.

Restoring Health Through Relaxation

Research suggests that relaxation techniques can be used to counteract the stress response, with significant health benefits. Regular relaxation can reduce blood cortisol levels, blood pressure, cholesterol, and blood glucose.

Clinical trials show that relaxation can reduce headaches, pain, anxiety, and menopausal symptoms. At the same time, it can enhance healing, immune cell response, concentration, and feelings of well-being. It has even shown to improve fertility rates in infertile women.

Research done in the 1970s by Dr. Herbert Benson of Harvard University began to explore the relationship between mental techniques and physiological effects. Benson studied people who participated in transcendental meditation. He coined the term "the relaxation response," which is defined as "a calm state brought about by sitting quietly and repeating a sound, words, or muscular activity over and over. When everyday thoughts intrude, the person passively disregards them and returns to the repetition." The relaxation response reflects a physiological state brought about by reducing stress and calming the mind.

The following effects are the result of the relaxation response:

- Reduced blood pressure
- Reduced heart rate
- Slower breathing rate
- Restoration of blood flow to the extremities
- Reduction in perspiration
- Release of muscular tension

When you look at the results of the relaxation response and compare them with the list at the beginning of the chapter, it's easy to see how relaxation counteracts the stress response and restores the body to a state of balance.

As a result of numerous studies in this area, relaxation techniques are used to help people with problems such as hypertension and cardiac arrhythmias, among others. While these skills are useful for people who are managing chronic disease, they are also valuable for promoting health and preventing stress-related illnesses. Make time to explore and learn techniques that help you relax.

ESSENTIAL

Researchers have observed that people who learn effective stress-management techniques are much more successful at achieving long-lasting behavioral change in the areas of improved nutrition, smoking cessation, increased physical activity, and weight management.

Relaxation and Deep Breathing

One of the easiest ways to achieve relaxation is to engage in deep, mindful breathing exercises. This can help trigger the relaxation response. This type of exercise is easy to learn, fast to perform, and requires no equipment. As you continue to explore other methods of relaxation, use the following breathing exercise to help you ease tensions and restore your sense of balance and calm. It will do the health of your body, mind, and spirit a world of good. As you emerge from your restorative relaxation time, remind yourself that you have the power to create your own health and enjoy all that life has to offer to you.

A Simple Breathing Exercise

This exercise is an excellent introduction to relaxation and meditation techniques. It increases self-awareness and body awareness. A two- to three-minute "breathing break" during the day is very restorative. To perform this simple exercise, sit or lie comfortably with your hands resting in your lap. Relax your muscles and close your eyes.

Make no effort to control your breath, simply breathe naturally. As you breathe in and out, focus your attention on the breath and how the body moves with each inhalation and exhalation.

Take a few moments to focus inward. Notice the movement of your body as you breathe. Observe your inhalation and exhalation. Pay particular attention to how the breath moves your body. Observe your chest, shoulders, rib cage, and belly. Notice subtleties such as whether the chest or belly rises with inhalation and how your body responds to exhalation. Don't try to control your breath, simply focus your attention on it. This singular focus brings you into the present moment and into the immediate experience of your body. It often results in slower, deeper breaths that further relax your body. Continue for two to three minutes and then gently open your eyes. Over time, you can lengthen the period of relaxation, if you prefer.

Restoring Life Through Meditation

For centuries, many have used meditation to reduce stress in their lives. The act of meditation is similar to relaxation in the attempt to let go of stressful thoughts. The key difference between meditation and relaxation is that during relaxation, one tries to passively empty the mind, while meditation represents active focus on certain thoughts through abandoning other thoughts.

Numerous studies have shown that meditation, like relaxation, improves health and mood. Meditation is also known to improve cognition and focus. Meditation produces many of the same physiologic changes as the relaxation response. Because of meditation's differences in practice of intense focus rather than lack of focus, meditation can better serve those who have difficulty emptying their mind and decompressing. Meditation can also be complementary. Similar to how varied exercises can further help your body, the most stress reduction is likely obtained by incorporating various practices that reduce stress. Not only do you obtain the benefits of each practice, but as with using different physical exercises to continue to develop and motivate the body, using different mental practices can help you continue to develop and motivate the mind.

Practicing Meditation

The practice of meditation can seem complex, but the basic concept is quite simple. The key, like relaxation, exercise, eating healthier, or changing or creating any other habit, is that it takes practice.

To begin, though you can commence nearly any time at any place, the ideal setting is a quiet area, sitting comfortably. Sitting on the floor with your back straight tends to focus your attention further and is recommended but not necessary. Start to breathe in and out. Once in a rhythm, begin to focus your thoughts on an area of your choice. Make that as specific an area as possible. You can focus on a certain aspect of your life, your family, your work, your health, or just simply focus on your breathing, being in the present moment.

What then makes meditation challenging is the other thoughts that enter your head. You may start to drift or hear a lot of background noise in your own mind. Recognize those other thoughts, do not get frustrated, and let go of those thoughts, bringing yourself back to where you originally wished to focus. This might seem simple, but you are constantly barraged with thoughts and stimuli throughout the day. Going even sixty seconds without allowing some new thought or stimulus is surprisingly challenging. With practice, you will notice you are able to focus for longer and longer periods. As with exercise, the more you do, the better it is for your health.

The highest yield of meditation is when you start your day and shortly before going to bed. Set a goal to practice for at least five minutes. You can derive significant benefit from five minutes, but once you are able to meditate that long without significant thought interruption, you may choose to practice even longer.

The Overall Benefits to You

With relaxation and meditation, many people feel they cannot spare the five minutes to obtain the significant benefit. Those who practice relaxation and meditation, though, know that the several minutes they spend incorporating either practice into their daily routine adds much more time to their lives. You will find it easier to focus, making you more productive. You will sleep better, making you feel more rested and able to do more. By reducing your stress, you will improve your cholesterol, blood pressure, and blood sugar, and make you feel more able to tackle other aspects of your health. This will add years to your life and improve the quality of those years.

CHAPTER 13

Heart-Healthy Soup, Appetizer, and Side-Dish Recipes

Spring Asparagus Soup

In February, the first asparagus comes in with a taste of spring. This puréed soup can also be made with other vegetables, like sugar-snap peas or baby peas.

INGREDIENTS | SERVES 4

1 tablespoon olive oil
3 scallions, chopped
½ cup finely chopped sweet onion
1 clove garlic, minced
2 new potatoes, peeled and chopped
1 pound asparagus
4 cups Low-Sodium Chicken Broth (see recipe in this chapter)
1 tablespoon lemon juice
1 teaspoon lemon zest
1 tablespoon fresh thyme leaves
⅛ teaspoon white pepper
1 cup fat-free half-and-half

1. In a large soup pot, heat olive oil over medium heat. Add scallions, sweet onion, and garlic; cook and stir for 3 minutes.

2. Add potatoes; cook and stir for 5 minutes longer.

3. Snap the asparagus spears and discard ends. Chop asparagus into 1" pieces and add to pot along with broth. Bring to a boil, reduce heat, cover, and simmer for 10 minutes.

4. Using an immersion blender, purée the soup until smooth.

5. Add lemon juice, lemon zest, thyme, pepper, and half-and-half.

6. Heat until steaming, and serve. You can also serve this soup chilled. (Without an immersion blender, purée the soup in 4 batches in a blender or food processor, then return to the pot and continue with the recipe.)

♥ **PER SERVING** Calories: 201.50 | Fat: 6.04 g | Saturated fat: 1.52 g | Sodium: 182.69 mg | Cholesterol: 3.03 mg

Chicken Curry Apple Soup

This soup is delicately flavored, perfect for lunch on the porch. If you can't find fresh herbs, use dried; reduce the amount by two-thirds.

INGREDIENTS | SERVES 6

2 cups chopped cooked chicken breast

3 cups Low-Sodium Chicken Broth (see recipe in this chapter)

2 cups unsweetened apple juice

2 tablespoons lemon juice

1 tablespoon curry powder

2 Granny Smith apples, chopped

1 tablespoon fresh thyme leaves

1 teaspoon finely chopped rosemary leaves

⅛ teaspoon pepper

½ cup chopped celery leaves

1. In a large pot, combine all ingredients except for celery leaves.

2. Bring to a boil, then reduce heat, cover, and simmer for 10–14 minutes, or until apple is tender and chicken is hot.

3. Garnish each serving with celery leaves.

   ♥ **PER SERVING** Calories: 262.31 | Fat: 3.95 g | Saturated fat: 1.09 g | Sodium: 114.86 mg | Cholesterol: 59.50 mg

Cantaloupe-Melon Soup

This soup is light, cool, and refreshing. You can substitute other melons like Casaba, orange honeydew, or Santa Claus if you'd like.

INGREDIENTS | SERVES 4

1 cup cracked ice

4 cups chopped ripe cantaloupe

2 cups chopped honeydew melon

4 fresh mint leaves

1 (6-ounce) can pineapple-orange juice

⅛ teaspoon Tabasco sauce

1 tablespoon lime juice

¼ teaspoon salt

1. In a blender or food processor, combine ice, cantaloupe, melon, mint, and pineapple-orange juice; cover and blend or process until smooth.

2. Place in a serving bowl and add Tabasco sauce, lime juice, and salt.

3. Cover and chill for 2–3 hours before serving.

   ♥ **PER SERVING** Calories: 109.47 | Fat: 0.43 g | Saturated fat: 0.11 g | Sodium: 187.74 mg | Cholesterol: 0.0 mg

Ripening Melons

When you buy melons, be sure to choose those that are heavy, with a sweet smell and evenly webbed skin.

Cabbage-Tomato-Bean Chowder

Cabbage becomes sweet when cooked, and is a great complement to tender beans and tangy tomatoes. A tiny bit of sugar helps counteract the acid in the tomatoes.

INGREDIENTS | SERVES 4

1 tablespoon olive oil

1 onion, chopped

4 cloves garlic, minced

3 cups shredded green cabbage

1 (14-ounce) can no-salt diced tomatoes, undrained

1 (6-ounce) can no-salt tomato paste

2 cups Low-Sodium Chicken Broth (see recipe in this chapter)

1 teaspoon sugar

⅛ teaspoon white pepper

2 cups Beans for Soup (see recipe in this chapter)

⅓ cup fat-free half-and-half

1. In a large saucepan, heat olive oil over medium heat. Add onion and garlic; cook and stir until crisp-tender, about 4 minutes. Add cabbage; cook and stir for 3 minutes longer.

2. Add tomatoes, tomato paste, chicken broth, sugar, and pepper. Cook and stir until tomato paste dissolves in soup.

3. Stir in beans and bring to a simmer. Simmer for 10 minutes, then add half-and-half. Heat until the soup steams, and serve.

♥ **PER SERVING** Calories: 272.75 | Fat: 4.96 g | Saturated fat: 0.95 g | Sodium: 148.66 mg | Cholesterol: 1.01 mg

Red Lentil Soup

This is a great, hearty soup that freezes really well. Make an extra batch and freeze it for those days when you just don't feel like cooking.

INGREDIENTS | SERVES 4

2 tablespoons olive oil

4 cloves garlic, minced

1 cup chopped onion

2 tablespoons minced gingerroot

2 parsnips, peeled and chopped

3 carrots, peeled and chopped

2 cups vegetable broth

2 cups water

2 sprigs fresh thyme

1 cup red lentils

1. In a large soup pot, heat olive oil over medium heat. Add garlic and onion; cook and stir until crisp-tender.

2. Add gingerroot, parsnips, and carrots; cook for 2 minutes. Stir in vegetable broth, water, and thyme; bring to a boil. Reduce heat, cover, and simmer for 10 minutes.

3. Sort over lentils and wash thoroughly. Add lentils to pot and bring back to a simmer. Simmer for 15–25 minutes, or until lentils and vegetables are tender.

4. Remove the thyme stems and discard.

♥ **PER SERVING** Calories: 271.98 | Fat: 8.05 g | Saturated fat: 1.24 g | Sodium: 41.12 mg | Cholesterol: 0.0 mg

Corn Polenta Chowder

Turkey bacon helps reduce the fat in this excellent thick chowder, but it is high in salt, so no additional salt is needed.

INGREDIENTS | SERVES 6

2 strips turkey bacon

1 tablespoon olive oil

1 red onion, chopped

3 cloves garlic, minced

1 red bell pepper, chopped

2 jalapeño peppers, minced

2 Yukon Gold potatoes, chopped

5 cups Low-Sodium Chicken Broth (see recipe in this chapter), divided

⅓ cup cornmeal

2 tablespoons adobo sauce

2 (10-ounce) packages frozen corn, thawed

1 cup fat-free half-and-half

¼ cup chopped cilantro

⅛ teaspoon cayenne pepper

1. In a large soup pot, cook bacon until crisp. Remove from heat, crumble, and set aside.

2. To drippings remaining in pot, add olive oil, then onion and garlic; cook and stir until tender, about 5 minutes.

3. Stir in the bell peppers, jalapeños, potatoes, and 3 cups of the broth. Bring to a boil; reduce heat, cover, and simmer for 20 minutes, until the potatoes are tender.

4. In a small microwave-safe bowl, combine cornmeal and 1 cup chicken broth. Microwave on high for 2 minutes; remove, stir, then microwave for 2–4 minutes longer, or until mixture thickens.

5. Stir in adobo sauce and remaining 1 cup chicken broth. Add to soup along with corn. Simmer for another 10 minutes.

6. Add the half-and-half, cilantro, and pepper; stir well. Heat until steam rises, then sprinkle with reserved bacon; serve immediately.

♥ **PER SERVING** Calories: 276.10 | Fat: 6.03 g | Saturated fat: 1.42 g | Sodium: 184.32 mg | Cholesterol: 6.22 mg

Beans for Soup

Since beans and legumes are so full of fiber and are a great way to reduce cholesterol, you should eat lots of them. Unfortunately, canned beans are very high in sodium. Make up a batch of these beans and freeze them, then use instead of canned beans.

INGREDIENTS | **YIELDS 10 CUPS; SERVING SIZE 1 CUP**

1 pound dried beans
Water, as needed

Sodium in Canned Beans

A cup of canned beans, even after they have been rinsed and drained, contains about 300–500 mg of sodium. A cup of dried beans, cooked until tender, has about 7 mg of sodium. Let your slow cooker do the cooking, and dramatically reduce your sodium intake. Cooking a large batch of beans all at once makes them almost as convenient as canned.

1. Sort beans, rinse well, and drain.

2. Combine in a large pot with water to cover by 1".

3. Bring to a boil over high heat; cover pan, remove from heat, and let stand for 2 hours.

4. Place pot in refrigerator and let beans soak overnight.

5. In the morning, drain beans and rinse; drain again. Place in a 5–6-quart slow cooker with water to just cover.

6. Cover and cook on low for 8–10 hours, until beans are tender. Do not add salt or any other ingredient.

7. Package beans in 1 cup portions into freezer bags, including a bit of the cooking liquid in each bag. Seal, label, and freeze for up to 3 months.

8. To use, defrost in refrigerator overnight or open bag and microwave on defrost until beans begin thawing, then stir into soup to heat.

♥ **PER SERVING** Calories: 219.48 | Fat: 0.16 g | Saturated fat: 0.03 g | Sodium: 7.08 mg | Cholesterol: 0.0 mg

Mediterranean Fish-and-Bean Stew

This rich recipe is packed full of flavor, fiber, and nutrition. Serve it with a nice green salad and Oat-Bran Dinner Rolls (see Chapter 16) for a complete and hearty meal.

INGREDIENTS | SERVES 8

2 tablespoons olive oil

1 onion, chopped

1 fennel bulb, chopped, fronds reserved

4 cloves garlic, minced

¼ teaspoon salt

¼ teaspoon white pepper

1 teaspoon dried thyme leaves

4 cups Beans for Soup (see recipe in this chapter)

1 (14-ounce) can diced tomatoes, undrained

1 (6-ounce) can no-salt tomato paste

4 cups Low-Sodium Chicken Broth (see recipe in this chapter)

1 cup dry white wine

3 cups water

1½ pounds cod or haddock fillets

¼ cup chopped flat-leaf parsley

2 tablespoons chopped fennel fronds

1. In a large soup pot, heat olive oil over medium heat. Add onion, fennel, and garlic; cook and stir until crisp-tender, about 5 minutes. Sprinkle with salt, pepper, and thyme leaves.

2. Add remaining ingredients except for fish fillets, parsley, and fennel fronds. Bring to a boil, reduce heat, and simmer for 20 minutes.

3. Add fish fillets; simmer for 8–10 minutes, or until fish flakes and is opaque. Stir gently to break up fish. Sprinkle with parsley and fennel fronds and serve.

♥ **PER SERVING** Calories: 330.85 | Fat: 6.92 g | Saturated fat: 1.09 g | Sodium: 192.53 mg | Cholesterol: 45.50 mg

About Fennel

Fennel is a root vegetable with a spicy licorice taste. Both the bulb and the fronds are edible. To prepare, cut off the root end and the fronds. Remove outer layer of the bulb and discard; slice the flesh. Submerge in water to remove the sand and grit between the layers. Drain and slice or coarsely chop. The fronds are excellent as a garnish; rinse and chop.

Scandinavian Summer Fruit Soup

This is wonderful for a summer brunch. To make this a winter soup, use dried fruits like raisins and apricots. Each serving of soup gives you more than 100 percent of your daily requirement of vitamin C.

INGREDIENTS | SERVES 6

4 cups apple cider
1 cup cranberry juice
½ cup orange juice
¼ cup lemon juice
¼ cup sugar
¼ teaspoon salt
4 peaches, peeled and chopped
1 pint strawberries, chopped
2 pears, peeled and chopped
2 cinnamon sticks
½ teaspoon ground cardamom
1 bunch fresh mint
6 tablespoons low-fat sour cream

1. Make the soup the day before serving. In a large bowl, combine apple cider, cranberry juice, orange juice, lemon juice, sugar, and salt.

2. Place half of the peaches, strawberries, and pears in a food processor or blender. Add 1 cup of the apple cider mixture and blend or process until smooth.

3. Add to apple cider mixture along with remaining ingredients except mint and sour cream. Cover and chill for at least 8 hours.

4. Remove cinnamon sticks and stir soup. Spoon soup into chilled bowls and garnish with mint and sour cream.

♥ **PER SERVING** Calories: 241.46 | Fat: 2.49 g | Saturated fat: 1.19 g | Sodium: 111.65 mg | Cholesterol: 5.85 mg

Low-Sodium Beef Broth

Even low-sodium varieties of canned beef broth have large amounts of sodium, about 400 mg per cup. This rich broth has hardly any sodium, but it does have lots of flavor.

INGREDIENTS | YIELDS 10 CUPS

3 pounds soup bones
1 pound beef shank
4 carrots, cut into 1" chunks
2 onions, chopped
2 tablespoons olive oil
2 bay leaves
5 cloves garlic, crushed
5 peppercorns
8 cups water

Making Broth

The secrets to making a rich broth include thoroughly browning the bones and vegetables and letting the broth simmer a long time. You can also clarify the broth; when the fat has been removed, bring the broth to a boil with the shell of an egg. Simmer for 5 minutes, then strain the broth through several layers of cheesecloth or a coffee strainer.

1. Preheat oven to 400°F. In a large roasting pan, place soup bones, beef shank, carrots, and onions. Drizzle with olive oil and toss to coat. Roast for 2 hours, or until bones and vegetables are brown.

2. Place roasted bones and vegetables along with bay leaves, garlic, and peppercorns in a 5–6-quart slow cooker. Pour 1 cup water into roasting pan and scrape up brown bits; add to slow cooker. Pour remaining water into slow cooker. Cover and cook on low for 8–9 hours.

3. Strain broth into a large bowl; discard solids. Cover broth and refrigerate overnight. In the morning, remove fat solidified on surface and discard. Pour broth into freezer containers, seal, label, and freeze up to 3 months.

4. To use, defrost in refrigerator overnight.

♥ **PER SERVING** Calories: 31.45 | Fat: 0.88 g | Saturated fat: 0.29 g | Sodium: 15.65 mg | Cholesterol: 8.85 mg

Low-Sodium Chicken Broth

Browning the chicken before making stock adds rich flavor and deepens the color.

INGREDIENTS | YIELDS 8 CUPS;
SERVING SIZE 1 CUP

2 tablespoons olive oil

3 pounds cut-up chicken

2 onions, chopped

5 cloves garlic, minced

4 carrots, sliced

4 stalks celery, sliced

1 tablespoon peppercorns

1 bay leaf

6 cups water

2 tablespoons lemon juice

1. In a large skillet, heat the olive oil over medium heat. Add the chicken, skin-side down, and cook until browned, about 8–10 minutes. Place chicken in 5–6-quart slow cooker.

2. Add onions and garlic to drippings in skillet; cook and stir for 2–3 minutes, scraping bottom of skillet.

3. Add to slow cooker along with remaining ingredients except lemon juice. Cover and cook on low for 8–9 hours.

4. Strain broth into a large bowl. Remove meat from chicken; refrigerate or freeze for another use. Cover broth and refrigerate overnight. In the morning, remove fat solidified on surface and discard. Stir in lemon juice. Pour broth into freezer containers, seal, label, and freeze up to 3 months.

5. To use, defrost in refrigerator overnight.

♥ **PER SERVING** Calories: 82.89 | Fat: 5.22 g | Saturated fat: 0.92 mg | Sodium: 39.09 mg | Cholesterol: 17.86 mg

Three-Bean Chili

Chili without meat is still rich and satisfying. If you love hot food,
use habanero peppers instead of the jalapeños.

INGREDIENTS | SERVES 6

1 cup dried black beans
1 cup dried kidney beans
1 cup dried pinto beans
2 jalapeño peppers, minced
2 onions, chopped
4 cloves garlic, minced
4 cups water
4 cups Low-Sodium Beef Broth (see recipe in this chapter), divided
2 (14-ounce) cans low-sodium diced tomatoes, undrained
1 (6-ounce) can low-sodium tomato paste
⅛ teaspoon pepper

1. Pick over beans and rinse well; drain and place in a large bowl. Cover with water and let stand overnight. In the morning, drain and rinse the beans and place them into a 4–5-quart slow cooker.

2. Add peppers, onions, garlic, water, and 3 cups broth to the slow cooker. Stir well. Cover and cook on low for 8 hours, or until beans are tender.

3. Add canned tomatoes to slow cooker.

4. In small bowl, combine remaining 1 cup broth with the tomato paste; stir with whisk to dissolve the tomato paste.

5. Add to slow cooker along with pepper. Cover and cook on low for 1–2 hours longer, or until chili is thick.

♥ **PER SERVING** Calories: 326.20 | Fat: 1.50 g | Saturated fat: 0.36 g | Sodium: 64.96 mg | Cholesterol: 4.42 mg

Steamer Clams in Ginger Sauce

This recipe is an excellent choice to serve during summer cocktail parties, or at your next beach barbecue.

INGREDIENTS | **SERVES 28**

2 teaspoons Bragg Liquid Aminos

1 teaspoon lemon juice

¼ cup spring onions, very thinly sliced

1 teaspoon white rice wine vinegar

4 teaspoons apple juice

1 teaspoon ground ginger

¼ teaspoon Oriental mustard powder

4 cloves garlic, minced or 1 teaspoon garlic powder

1 teaspoon dried green onion flakes

¼ teaspoon granulated sugar

1 (15-ounce) Gordon's Chesapeake Classics Cocktail Clams (Steamer Size), drained

1 large cucumber

1. In a bowl, combine all ingredients except the steamer clams and cucumber. Add the drained clams; toss to mix.

2. Wash and slice the cucumber. Arrange the cucumber slices on a platter; place a clam atop each slice. Chill until ready to serve.

♥ **PER SERVING** Calories: 10.19 | Fat: 0.02 g | Saturated fat: 0.00 g | Sodium: 88.51 mg | Cholesterol: 2.50 mg

Super Spicy Salsa

Salsa can be used in so many ways. It's fabulous as a garnish for chili or grilled chicken.

INGREDIENTS | **YIELDS 3 CUPS; SERVING SIZE ¼ CUP**

2 jalapeño peppers, minced

1 habanero pepper, minced

1 green bell pepper, minced

4 cloves garlic, minced

1 red onion, chopped

5 ripe tomatoes, chopped

3 tablespoons lemon juice

¼ teaspoon salt

⅛ teaspoon white pepper

¼ cup chopped fresh cilantro

1. In a large bowl, combine jalapeños, habanero, bell pepper, garlic, red onion, and tomatoes.

2. In a small bowl, combine lemon juice, salt, and pepper; stir to dissolve salt. Add to tomato mixture along with cilantro.

3. Cover and refrigerate for 3–4 hours before serving.

♥ **PER SERVING** Calories: 25.23 | Fat: 0.21 g | Saturated fat: 0.05 g | Sodium: 53.25 mg | Cholesterol: 0.0 mg

Sweet Stuff Guacamole Dip

Apple cider vinegar and apple juice add a sweet tang in this guacamole recipe. Try it on tacos and burritos, too!

INGREDIENTS | SERVES 16

1 avocado, peeled and pitted

1½ teaspoons apple cider vinegar

1 clove garlic

1 teaspoon Bragg Liquid Aminos

½ teaspoon Lea & Perrins Worcestershire sauce

2 teaspoons extra-virgin olive oil

2 tablespoons apple juice

½ cup plain nonfat yogurt

1 teaspoon fresh lemon juice

1. In a blender or food processor, process all ingredients until smooth.

2. Serve with unsalted tortilla chips.

♥ **PER SERVING** Calories: 31.50 | Fat: 2.44 g | Saturated Fat: 0.39 g | Sodium: 29.56 mg | Cholesterol: 0.39 mg

Roasted Garlic and Red Pepper Hummus

This recipe is a twist on a delicious party classic. The roasted garlic and roasted red peppers add sweet flavor without being overpowering.

INGREDIENTS | SERVES 32; SERVING SIZE 1 TABLESPOON

2 cloves Roasted Garlic (see recipe in this chapter)

2 cups cooked no-salt-added garbanzo beans, drained

⅓ cup tahini

⅓ cup lemon juice

½ cup chopped roasted red peppers

¼ teaspoon dried basil

Freshly ground black pepper, to taste

1. In a food processor, combine the garlic, garbanzo beans, tahini, lemon juice, chopped red peppers, and basil. Process until the mixture is smooth.

2. Season to taste with freshly ground pepper. Transfer the hummus to a covered bowl and chill until ready to serve.

♥ **PER SERVING** Calories: 32.57 | Fat: 1.47 g | Saturated fat: 0.20 g | Sodium: 2.67 mg | Cholesterol: 0.00 mg

Open-Face Wild Mushroom Wontons

These delicate, delicious wontons are a gourmet addition to your standard party fare. Your guests won't believe they're healthy!

INGREDIENTS | SERVES 24

1 tablespoon olive or canola oil

1 tablespoon unsalted butter

½ cup sliced shallots

½ teaspoon freshly ground black pepper

¾ pound assorted wild mushrooms (such as chanterelle, wood ear, shiitake, morel), cleaned, stemmed, and thinly sliced

¾ cup water

¾ teaspoon Minor's Low Sodium Chicken Base

¼ cup instant nonfat dry milk

½ cup ricotta cheese

½ teaspoon herbal seasoning blend of your choice

24 wonton wrappers

Spectrum Naturals Extra Virgin Olive Spray Oil, to taste

2 tablespoons grated Parmesan cheese

Go Natural!

Most processed foods have high sodium levels that result from the combination of salt added to the food and the high sodium content of the preservatives. Do all you can to keep the foods you eat as close to natural as possible.

1. Preheat oven to 375°F.

2. In a large, heavy nonstick skillet, heat the oil and melt the butter over medium-high heat. Add the shallots and cook, stirring, for 1 minute.

3. Add the pepper and mushrooms; sauté until the mushrooms become soft and most of the mushroom liquid is evaporated, about 8 minutes.

4. Add the water and heat until it begins to boil. Dissolve the Minor's base in the water.

5. Reduce heat and add the nonfat dry milk, whisking to combine with the mushroom mixture.

6. Add the ricotta cheese and herbal seasoning, and mix to combine; cook until heated through. Remove from heat.

7. Line a baking sheet with nonstick aluminum foil. Prepare the wonton wrappers by lightly spraying 1 side of each with the spray oil. Place sprayed-side down on the foil. Evenly divide the mushroom mixture, placing a spoonful on each wonton wrapper. Top the mushroom mixture with the grated cheese.

8. Bake for 8–10 minutes, or until the wontons are brown and crunchy and the cheese is melted and bubbly.

♥ **PER SERVING** Calories: 54.23 | Fat: 2.06 g | Saturated fat: 0.92 g | Sodium: 72.42 mg | Cholesterol: 5.12 mg

Roasted Garlic

Believe it or not, roasted garlic is a fabulous treat eaten all by itself. You can also spread it on bread, mash it into some low-fat cream cheese for a sandwich spread, or add to sauces.

INGREDIENTS | SERVES 6

1 head garlic
2 teaspoons olive oil
Pinch salt
1 teaspoon lemon juice

Freezing Roasted Garlic

Make a lot of Roasted Garlic. When the garlic is cool, squeeze the cloves out of the papery covering; discard the covering. Place the garlic in a small bowl and work into a paste. Freeze in ice cube trays until solid, then place in heavy-duty freezer bags, label, and freeze up to 3 months. To use, just cut off the amount you want and thaw in fridge.

1. Preheat oven to 400°F.

2. Peel off some of the outer skins from the garlic head, leaving the head whole. Cut off the top ½" of the garlic head; discard top.

3. Place on a square of heavy-duty aluminum foil, cut-side up. Drizzle with the olive oil, making sure the oil runs into the cloves. Sprinkle with salt and lemon juice.

4. Wrap garlic in foil, covering completely. Place on a baking sheet and roast for 40–50 minutes, or until garlic is very soft and golden brown.

5. Let cool for 15 minutes, then serve or use in recipes.

♥ **PER SERVING** Calories: 32.10 | Fat: 1.56 g | Saturated fat: 0.22 g | Sodium: 28.00 mg | Cholesterol: 0.0 mg

Sweet Pea Guacamole

Using sweet peas instead of avocados significantly reduces the amount of fat in this dip. Keep the jalapeño seeds in if you like extra heat.

INGREDIENTS | SERVES 8; SERVING SIZE ⅔ CUP

3 tablespoons extra-virgin olive oil

2 tablespoons fresh lime juice

2 tablespoons minced fresh coriander

2 jalapeño peppers, seeded and minced

½ teaspoon ground cumin

½ teaspoon ground coriander

½ teaspoon ground black pepper

1 (16-ounce) package Cascadian Farm Organic frozen Garden Peas, cooked without salt and drained

2 plum tomatoes, peeled, seeded, and diced

1 small red onion, finely diced

Honey or jalapeño jelly, to taste (optional)

1. In a food processor, combine the oil, lime juice, coriander leaves, peppers, spices, and black pepper; process until smooth.

2. Add the peas. Pulse a few times to chop the peas and combine with the other ingredients.

3. Use a spatula to scrape the mixture into a serving bowl.

4. Stir in the tomato and onion. Check seasoning and adjust if necessary, adding some honey or jalapeño jelly if a touch of sweetness is necessary to mellow the hotness of the peppers.

♥ **PER SERVING** Calories: 102.38 | Fat: 5.15 g | Saturated fat: 0.69 g | Sodium: 66.78 mg | Cholesterol: 0.00 mg

Hidden Sodium

Frozen peas are sorted by size in saltwater baths. As a result, they'll already have a higher sodium content than fresh ones. If you use frozen peas, make sure you use a no-additional-salt-added variety. Using the worst-case scenario formula, the nutritional analysis for the Sweet Pea Guacamole recipe was calculated using the named brand frozen peas that have 95 mg sodium per ⅔ cup serving; other brands may vary.

Honey-Almond Spread

This spread is delicious on whole-wheat bagels or English muffins.
Try it with crackers or chopped vegetables, too.

INGREDIENTS | SERVES 32; SERVING SIZE 1 TABLESPOON

2 tablespoons fresh orange juice

½ cup chopped raisins

1 tablespoon honey

4 ounces cream cheese

½ cup plain nonfat yogurt

¼ cup chopped Honey-Spiced Almonds (see recipe in this chapter)

1. Mix together the orange juice and raisins; set aside.

2. In a small bowl, mix together the honey, cream cheese, and yogurt.

3. Stir the chopped raisins-orange juice mixture and almonds into the cream cheese mixture.

4. Cover, and chill in the refrigerator until ready to serve.

♥ **PER SERVING** Calories: 26.65 | Fat: 1.47 g | Saturated fat: 0.82 g | Sodium: 13.53 mg | Cholesterol: 4.05 mg

Honey-Spiced Almonds

Serve this snack at your next holiday gathering. Your guests will
love a change from the traditional party peanuts!

INGREDIENTS | SERVES 12

2 tablespoons unsalted butter

½ teaspoon cinnamon

⅛ teaspoon ground cloves

⅛ teaspoon ground ginger

½ cup honey

½ teaspoon orange zest

3 cups raw almonds

1. Put the butter, spices, honey, and orange zest in a large microwave-safe bowl. Microwave on high for 1 minute, or until the butter is melted. Stir well to combine.

2. Add the almonds to the honey mixture; stir well to combine. Microwave on high for 3 minutes; stir well. Microwave on high for another 3 minutes; stir.

3. Spread the nuts on a nonstick foil-lined baking sheet to cool. Be careful—the mixture will be very hot!

♥ **PER SERVING** Calories: 98.59 | Fat: 6.97 g | Saturated fat: 1.06 g | Sodium: 0.53 mg | Cholesterol: 2.59 mg

Pissaladiere (Onion Tart)

This recipe may take a bit longer to prepare than your standard appetizer, but the results are worth it. The mix of herbs and spices compliment the sweet onions and Parmesan for a perfect blend of flavors in every bite.

INGREDIENTS | SERVES 24

¼ teaspoon dried lemon granules, crushed

¼ teaspoon mustard powder

1 tablespoon water

1 tablespoon extra-virgin olive oil

2 large sweet onions, thinly sliced

4 medium-size cloves garlic, finely chopped

1 fresh bay leaf

¼ teaspoon dried thyme, crushed

2 teaspoons dried parsley, crushed

¼ teaspoon freshly ground black pepper

Pinch dried red pepper flakes

½ recipe Basic White Bread dough (see Chapter 16)

2 tablespoons grated Parmesan cheese

1. Preheat the oven to 450°F with a rack set in the center position.

2. Add the lemon granules and mustard powder to a small microwave-safe bowl or coffee cup; spoon the water and oil over the top. Microwave on high for 30 seconds; cover with plastic wrap, and set aside.

3. Add onion, garlic, and bay leaf to a microwave-safe bowl. Cover and microwave on high for 4 minutes. Turn the bowl and microwave on high for an additional 3 minutes.

4. Discard the bay leaf and mix in the thyme, parsley, pepper, and red pepper flakes; cover and set aside.

5. Treat a 13" × 18" rimmed baking sheet with spray oil. Place the dough on a lightly floured surface and roll into a 13" × 18" rectangle; transfer to the baking pan. Cover with a damp cotton towel or plastic wrap and let rest for 30 minutes to rise.

6. Prick the dough all over with the tines of a fork. Uncover the lemon granules mixture and whisk with a fork. Brush the mixture evenly over the dough.

7. Stir the Parmesan cheese into the cooked onion mixture; spread the mixture evenly over the prepared dough. Bake for 12 minutes.

8. Rotate the pan; bake until the crust is cooked through and the edges are lightly browned.

9. Remove from oven and transfer the tart to a serving board. Slice and serve warm or at room temperature.

♥ **PER SERVING** Calories: 55.76 | Fat: 1.38 g | Saturated fat: 0.25 g | Sodium: 56.86 mg | Cholesterol: 0.33 mg

Carbonara Tart

This Italian-inspired tart will be a hit at your next dinner party.
Try adding some fresh chopped basil for extra flavor.

INGREDIENTS | SERVES 24

¾ teaspoon Minor's Bacon Base

1 tablespoon water

1 tablespoon extra-virgin olive oil

2 large sweet onions, thinly sliced

4 medium-size cloves garlic, finely chopped

1 fresh bay leaf

¼ teaspoon dried thyme, crushed

2 teaspoons dried parsley, crushed

¼ teaspoon freshly ground black pepper

Pinch dried red pepper flakes

½ recipe Basic White Bread dough (see Chapter 16)

4 eggs, beaten

2 tablespoons grated Parmesan cheese

1. Preheat the oven to 450°F with a rack set in the center position.

2. Add the bacon base to a small microwave-safe bowl or coffee cup; spoon the water and oil over the top. Microwave on high for 30 seconds; cover with plastic wrap and set aside.

3. Add onion, garlic, and bay leaf to a microwave-safe bowl. Cover and microwave on high for 4 minutes. Turn the bowl and microwave on high for an additional 3 minutes.

4. Discard the bay leaf and mix in the thyme, parsley, pepper, and red pepper flakes; cover and set aside.

5. Treat a 13" × 18" rimmed baking sheet with spray oil. Place the dough on a lightly floured surface and roll the dough into a 13" × 18" rectangle; transfer to the baking pan. Cover with a damp cotton towel or plastic wrap and let rest for 30 minutes to rise.

6. Prick the dough all over with the tines of a fork. Uncover the bacon base mixture and whisk with a fork. Brush the mixture evenly over the dough.

7. Stir the eggs and Parmesan cheese into the cooked onion mixture; spread the mixture evenly over the prepared dough. Bake for 12 minutes. Rotate the pan and bake until the crust is cooked through and the edges are lightly browned, about 12 minutes more.

8. Remove from oven and transfer the tart to a serving board. Slice and serve warm or at room temperature.

♥ **PER SERVING** Calories: 68.84 | Fat: 2.27 g | Saturated fat: 0.53 g | Sodium: 95.61 mg | Cholesterol: 35.80 mg

Greek Onion Tart

The Kalamata olives, feta, and nutmeg add Mediterranean flare to this outrageously delicious onion tart.

INGREDIENTS | SERVES 24

¼ teaspoon dried lemon granules, crushed

¼ teaspoon mustard powder

1 tablespoon water

1 tablespoon extra-virgin olive oil

2 large sweet onions, thinly sliced

4 medium-size cloves garlic, finely chopped

1 fresh bay leaf

¼ teaspoon dried thyme, crushed

2 teaspoons dried parsley, crushed

¼ teaspoon freshly ground black pepper

Pinch dried red pepper flakes

½ recipe Basic White Bread dough (see Chapter 16)

12 pitted Kalamata olives, sliced

1 ounce feta cheese, crumbled

Freshly ground nutmeg (optional)

1. Preheat the oven to 450°F with a rack set in the center position.

2. Add the lemon granules and mustard powder to a small microwave-safe bowl or coffee cup; spoon the water and oil over the top. Microwave on high for 30 seconds; cover with plastic wrap and set aside.

3. Add the onion, garlic, and bay leaf to a microwave-safe bowl. Cover and microwave on high for 4 minutes. Turn the bowl and microwave on high for an additional 3 minutes. Carefully remove the cover. Discard the bay leaf and mix in the thyme, parsley, pepper, and red pepper flakes; cover and set aside.

4. Treat a 13" × 18" rimmed baking sheet with spray oil. Place the dough on a lightly floured surface and roll dough into a 13" × 18" rectangle; transfer the dough to the baking pan. Cover with a damp cotton towel or plastic wrap and let rest for 30 minutes to rise.

5. Prick the dough all over with the tines of a fork. Uncover the lemon granules mixture and whisk with a fork. Brush the mixture evenly over the dough.

6. Stir the olives into the cooked onion mixture; spread the mixture evenly over the prepared dough. Sprinkle the feta cheese over the top of the onions.

7. Bake for 12 minutes. Rotate the pan and bake until the crust is cooked through and the edges are lightly browned.

8. Remove from oven and transfer the tart to a serving board. Slice and serve warm; grate nutmeg over the top, if desired.

♥ **PER SERVING** Calories: 64.48 | Fat: 2.26 g | Saturated fat: 0.35 g | Sodium: 177.29 mg | Cholesterol: 1.05 mg

Onion Dip

Here's a fresh take on a party classic! Serve it with plenty of veggies for dipping.

INGREDIENTS | SERVES 16

2 teaspoons onion powder

½ teaspoon dried green onion flakes

⅛ teaspoon dried granulated roasted garlic

⅛ teaspoon dried or freeze-dried chopped chives

⅛ teaspoon dried parsley

⅛ teaspoon celery seed

⅛ teaspoon dry mustard

½ cup plain nonfat yogurt

4 ounces cream cheese, at room temperature

1 tablespoon Hellmann's or Best Foods Real Mayonnaise

1 teaspoon Lea & Perrins Worcestershire sauce

2–3 drops hot pepper sauce (optional)

Freshly ground pink or black pepper, to taste (optional)

In a small bowl, add all ingredients; mix to combine. Cover and refrigerate until needed.

♥ **PER SERVING** Calories: 33.51 | Fat: 2.79 g | Saturated fat: 1.61 g | Sodium: 33.54 mg | Cholesterol: 8.19 mg

CHAPTER 14

Heart-Healthy Meat and Poultry Main-Dish Recipes

Chicken Breasts with Salsa

Whole-grain cereal provides lots of folic acid, which helps reduce homocysteine levels. It makes a nice crunchy coating on chicken breasts.

INGREDIENTS | **SERVES 4**

2 tablespoons lime juice, divided

1 egg white

1 cup whole-grain cereal, crushed

1 teaspoon dried thyme leaves

¼ teaspoon pepper

4 (4-ounce) boneless, skinless chicken breasts

1 cup Super Spicy Salsa (see Chapter 13)

1 jalapeño pepper, minced

1. Preheat the oven to 375°F. Line a cookie sheet with parchment paper and set aside.

2. In a small bowl, combine 1 tablespoon lime juice and egg white; beat until frothy.

3. On a shallow plate, combine crushed cereal, thyme, and pepper.

4. Dip chicken into egg white mixture, then into cereal mixture to coat. Place on prepared cookie sheet.

5. Bake for 20–25 minutes, or until chicken is thoroughly cooked and coating is crisp.

6. In a small saucepan, combine remaining 1 tablespoon lime juice, salsa, and jalapeño pepper. Heat through, stirring occasionally. Serve with chicken.

♥ **PER SERVING** Calories: 264.05 | Fat: 4.43 g | Saturated fat: 1.18 g | Sodium: 146.85 mg | Cholesterol: 90.36 mg

Sautéed Chicken with Roasted Garlic Sauce

When roasted, garlic turns sweet and nutty. Combined with tender sautéed chicken, this makes a memorable meal.

INGREDIENTS | SERVES 4

1 head Roasted Garlic (see Chapter 13)

⅓ cup Low-Sodium Chicken Broth (see Chapter 13)

½ teaspoon dried oregano leaves

¼ cup flour

⅛ teaspoon salt

⅛ teaspoon pepper

¼ teaspoon paprika

4 (4-ounce) boneless, skinless chicken breasts

2 tablespoons olive oil

Chicken and Cholesterol

Chicken is fairly high in cholesterol, but it's very low in saturated fat. The American Heart Association has boneless, skinless chicken breasts on its approved foods list, so you don't have to worry. If you are susceptible to cholesterol in food, reduce the serving size to 3 ounces per person.

1. In a small saucepan, squeeze garlic cloves from the skins and combine with broth and oregano.

2. On a shallow plate, combine flour, salt, pepper, and paprika. Dip chicken into this mixture to coat.

3. In a large skillet, heat 2 tablespoons olive oil. At the same time, place the saucepan with the garlic mixture over medium heat.

4. Add the chicken to the hot olive oil; cook for 5 minutes without moving. Then carefully turn chicken and cook for 4–7 minutes longer, until chicken is thoroughly cooked.

5. Stir garlic sauce with wire whisk until blended. Serve with the chicken.

♥ **PER SERVING** Calories: 267.01 | Fat: 7.78 g | Saturated fat: 1.65 g | Sodium: 158.61 mg | Cholesterol: 91.85 mg

Asian Chicken Stir-Fry

Yellow summer squash is a thin-skinned squash like zucchini. It has a mild, sweet flavor.

INGREDIENTS | SERVES 4

2 (5-ounce) boneless, skinless chicken breasts

½ cup Low-Sodium Chicken Broth (see Chapter 13)

1 tablespoon low-sodium soy sauce

1 tablespoon cornstarch

1 tablespoon sherry

2 tablespoons peanut oil

1 onion, sliced

3 cloves garlic, minced

1 tablespoon grated gingerroot

1 cup snow peas

½ cup canned sliced water chestnuts, drained

1 yellow summer squash, sliced

¼ cup chopped unsalted peanuts

1. Cut chicken into strips and set aside.

2. In a small bowl, combine broth, soy sauce, cornstarch, and sherry; set aside.

3. In a large skillet or wok, heat peanut oil over medium-high heat. Add chicken; stir-fry until almost cooked, about 3–4 minutes. Remove to plate.

4. Add onion, garlic, and gingerroot to skillet; stir-fry for 4 minutes longer.

5. Add snow peas, water chestnuts, and squash; stir-fry for 2 minutes longer.

6. Stir chicken broth mixture and add to skillet along with chicken. Stir-fry for 3–4 minutes longer, or until chicken is thoroughly cooked and sauce is thickened and bubbly. Sprinkle with peanuts and serve immediately.

♥ **PER SERVING** Calories: 252.42 | Fat: 12.42 g | Saturated fat: 2.06 g | Sodium: 202.04 mg | Cholesterol: 41.11 mg

Chicken Breasts with Mashed Beans

For a pretty presentation, divide the beans among plates and top with a sautéed chicken breast.

INGREDIENTS | SERVES 6

3 tablespoons olive oil, divided

1 onion, chopped

3 cloves garlic, minced

1 (14-ounce) can low-sodium cannellini beans

½ cup chopped flat-leaf parsley

½ teaspoon dried oregano leaves

1 teaspoon dried basil leaves

¼ cup grated Parmesan cheese

3 tablespoons flour

¼ teaspoon white pepper

6 (4-ounce) boneless, skinless chicken breasts

1. In a medium saucepan, heat 1 tablespoon olive oil and add onion and garlic. Cook and stir until tender, about 5 minutes.

2. Drain beans, rinse, and drain again. Add to saucepan along with parsley, oregano, and basil. Cook until hot, stirring frequently, about 5 minutes.

3. Using a potato masher, mash the bean mixture. Turn heat to very low.

4. On a shallow plate, combine Parmesan, flour, and pepper; mix well. Coat chicken on both sides with cheese mixture.

5. In a large skillet, heat remaining 2 tablespoons olive oil over medium heat.

6. Add chicken to skillet; cook for 5 minutes without moving. Carefully turn chicken and cook for 4–6 minutes, until thoroughly cooked. Serve with mashed beans.

♥ **PER SERVING** Calories: 316.30 | Fat: 10.55 g | Saturated fat: 2.56 g | Sodium: 133.71 mg | Cholesterol: 97.34 mg

Chicken Spicy Thai–Style

Peanut butter thickens the sauce and adds rich flavor to this easy stir-fry without adding any cholesterol.

INGREDIENTS | SERVES 4

2 tablespoons lime juice

1 tablespoon low-sodium soy sauce

½ cup Low-Sodium Chicken Broth (see Chapter 13)

¼ cup dry white wine

¼ cup natural peanut butter

2 tablespoons peanut oil

1 onion, chopped

4 cloves garlic, minced

3 (4-ounce) boneless, skinless chicken breasts, sliced

4 cups shredded Napa cabbage

1 cup shredded carrots

Natural Peanut Butter

Whenever possible, use natural peanut butter, not the regular kind found on store shelves. Read labels carefully. You'll notice that most regular peanut butter contains hydrogenated vegetable oil, which is a source of trans fat. The oil will separate out of the natural peanut butter as it stands; just stir it back in before using.

1. In a small bowl, combine lime juice, soy sauce, broth, wine, and peanut butter; mix with wire whisk until blended. Set aside.

2. In a wok or large skillet, heat peanut oil over medium-high heat. Add onion and garlic; stir-fry until crisp-tender, about 4 minutes.

3. Add chicken; stir-fry until almost cooked, about 3 minutes.

4. Add cabbage and carrots; stir-fry until cabbage begins to wilt, about 3–4 minutes longer.

5. Remove food from wok and return wok to heat. Add peanut butter mixture and bring to a simmer.

6. Return chicken and vegetables to wok; stir fry until sauce bubbles and thickens and chicken is thoroughly cooked, about 3–4 minutes. Serve immediately.

♥ **PER SERVING** Calories: 300.35 | Fat: 16.70 g | Saturated fat: 3.20 g | Sodium: 309.32 mg | Cholesterol: 51.56 mg

Chicken Breasts with New Potatoes

This easy one-dish meal has the best combination of flavors. Mustard adds a nice bit of spice to tender chicken and crisp potatoes.

INGREDIENTS | SERVES 6

12 small new red potatoes

2 tablespoons olive oil

⅛ teaspoon white pepper

4 cloves garlic, minced

1 teaspoon dried oregano leaves

2 tablespoons Dijon mustard

4 (4-ounce) boneless, skinless chicken breasts

1 cup cherry tomatoes

1. Preheat the oven to 400°F. Line a roasting pan with parchment paper and set aside. Scrub potatoes and cut each in half. Place in prepared pan.

2. In a small bowl, combine oil, pepper, garlic, oregano, and mustard; mix well. Drizzle half of this mixture over the potatoes; toss to coat. Roast for 20 minutes.

3. Cut chicken breasts into quarters. Remove pan from oven and add chicken to potato mixture. Using a spatula, mix potatoes and chicken together. Drizzle with remaining oil mixture. Return to oven and roast for 15 minutes longer.

4. Add tomatoes to pan. Roast for 5–10 minutes longer, or until potatoes are tender and browned and chicken is thoroughly cooked.

♥ **PER SERVING** Calories: 395.92 | Fat: 9.57 g | Saturated fat: 1.85 g | Sodium: 142.98 mg | Cholesterol: 61.23 mg

Chicken Poached in Tomato Sauce

Tarragon is a mild, licorice-tasting herb that pairs beautifully with chicken and tomatoes.

INGREDIENTS | SERVES 4

1 cup brown rice

2 cups water

2 tablespoons olive oil

1 onion, chopped

3 cloves garlic, minced

2 cups chopped plum tomatoes

½ teaspoon dried tarragon

¼ cup dry red wine

3 tablespoons no-salt tomato paste

1 cup Low-Sodium Chicken Broth (see Chapter 13)

⅛ teaspoon salt

⅛ teaspoon pepper

3 (5-ounce) boneless, skinless chicken thighs, sliced

Tomato Paste

If you don't use a whole can of tomato paste, you can freeze the rest for another use. Freeze the tomato paste in 1-tablespoon portions on a cookie sheet, then package into a freezer bag, label, and freeze for up to 3 months. To use, let stand at room temperature for 15 minutes, then use in recipe.

1. In a medium saucepan, combine rice and water; bring to a boil over high heat. Reduce heat to low, cover, and simmer for 30–40 minutes, or until rice is tender.

2. In a large saucepan, heat olive oil over medium heat. Add onion and garlic; cook and stir for 4 minutes, until crisp-tender.

3. Add tomatoes, tarragon, wine, tomato paste, chicken broth, salt, and pepper; bring to a simmer, stirring frequently.

4. Add chicken and bring back to a simmer. Cover pan, reduce heat to low, and poach chicken for 15–20 minutes, or until thoroughly cooked. Serve over hot cooked rice.

♥ **PER SERVING** Calories: 285.33 | Fat: 9.22 g | Saturated fat: 1.70 g | Sodium: 129.66 mg | Cholesterol: 61.80 mg

Hazelnut-Crusted Chicken Breasts

This super-quick dish is perfect for a last-minute dinner. Serve with a spinach salad and some crisp breadsticks.

INGREDIENTS | SERVES 2

2 (4-ounce) boneless, skinless chicken breasts
Pinch salt
Pinch pepper
1 tablespoon Dijon mustard
1 egg white
⅓ cup chopped hazelnuts
1 tablespoon olive oil

1. Place chicken between 2 sheets of waxed paper. Pound, starting at center of chicken, until ¼" thick. Sprinkle chicken with salt and pepper. Spread each side of chicken with some of the mustard.

2. Beat egg white until foamy. Dip chicken into egg white, then into hazelnuts, pressing to coat both sides.

3. In a skillet, heat olive oil over medium heat. Add chicken; cook for 3 minutes without moving. Turn and cook for 1–3 minutes on second side, until chicken is thoroughly cooked and nuts are toasted. Serve immediately.

♥ **PER SERVING** Calories: 276.64 | Fat: 16.02 g | Saturated fat: 1.88 g | Sodium: 266.25 mg | Cholesterol: 65.77 mg

Tomatoes with Chicken Mousse

Serve this elegant dish for a ladies' lunch along with a fruit salad and Lite Creamy Cheesecake (see Chapter 16) for dessert.

INGREDIENTS | SERVES 4

1 cup diced cooked chicken
¼ cup minced red onion
1 tablespoon chopped fresh chives
1 tablespoon fresh rosemary, minced
⅓ cup low-fat yogurt
¼ cup low-fat mayonnaise
1 tablespoon lime juice
½ cup chopped celery
4 large ripe tomatoes

1. In a blender or food processor, combine all ingredients except celery and tomatoes. Blend or process until smooth. Stir in celery.

2. Cut the tops off the tomatoes and scoop out the insides, leaving a ⅓" shell. Turn upside down on paper towels and let drain for 10 minutes.

3. Fill tomatoes with the chicken mixture and top each with the tomato top. Cover and chill for 2–3 hours before serving.

♥ **PER SERVING** Calories: 169.29 | Fat: 7.01 g | Saturated fat: 1.41 g | Sodium: 167.31 mg | Cholesterol: 30.98 mg

Texas Barbecue Chicken Thighs

*Make a double batch of this fabulous barbecue sauce all by itself in your
slow cooker and freeze it in ¼-cup portions to use anytime.*

INGREDIENTS | SERVES 6

2 tablespoons olive oil

1 onion, chopped

4 cloves garlic, minced

1 jalapeño pepper, minced

¼ cup orange juice

1 tablespoon low-sodium soy sauce

2 tablespoons apple-cider vinegar

2 tablespoons brown sugar

2 tablespoons Dijon mustard

1 (14-ounce) can crushed tomatoes, undrained

½ teaspoon cumin

1 tablespoon chili powder

¼ teaspoon pepper

6 (4-ounce) boneless, skinless chicken thighs

1. In a small skillet, heat olive oil over medium heat. Add onion and garlic; cook and stir until crisp-tender, about 4 minutes.

2. Place in a 3–4 quart slow cooker; add jalapeño, orange juice, soy sauce, vinegar, brown sugar, mustard, tomatoes, cumin, chili powder, and pepper.

3. Add chicken to the sauce, pushing chicken into the sauce to completely cover.

4. Cover and cook on low for 8–10 hours, or until chicken is thoroughly cooked.

♥ **PER SERVING** Calories: 236.53 | Fat: 9.30 g | Saturated fat: 1.79 g | Sodium: 277.24 mg | Cholesterol: 94.12 mg

Turkey Cutlets Florentine

*The word "Florentine" on a menu means spinach. This deep-green
leaf is full of antioxidants and fiber. And it's delicious, too!*

INGREDIENTS | SERVES 6

1 egg white, beaten
½ cup dry bread crumbs
⅛ teaspoon white pepper
2 tablespoons grated Parmesan cheese
6 (4-ounce) turkey cutlets
2 tablespoons olive oil
2 cloves minced garlic
2 (8-ounce) bags fresh baby spinach
⅛ teaspoon ground nutmeg
⅓ cup shredded Jarlsberg cheese

Cheeses

You can use low-fat or nonfat cheeses, but
they really don't have much flavor. Try using
smaller amounts of very sharply flavored
cheeses instead. Use extra-sharp Cheddar
instead of Colby; Gruyère instead of Swiss;
and Cotija instead of Parmesan. Grating or
shredding cheese will also enhance the flavor and allow you to use less.

1. In a shallow bowl, place egg white; beat until foamy.

2. On a shallow plate, combine bread crumbs, pepper,
   and Parmesan; mix well.

3. Place turkey cutlets between waxed paper and pound
   to ⅛" thickness, if necessary. Dip cutlets into egg white,
   then into breadcrumb mixture to coat.

4. In a large saucepan, heat olive oil over medium-high
   heat. Add turkey; cook for 4 minutes. Carefully turn and
   cook for 4–6 minutes longer, until thoroughly cooked.
   Remove to serving plate and cover with foil to keep
   warm.

   Add garlic to drippings remaining in pan; cook and stir
   for 1 minute. Add spinach and nutmeg; cook and stir
   until spinach wilts, about 4–5 minutes.

5. Add the Jarlsberg, top with the turkey; cover, and
   remove from heat. Let stand for 2 minutes to melt
   cheese, then serve.

♥ **PER SERVING** Calories: 258.57 | Fat: 9.19 g | Saturated fat:
2.15 g | Sodium: 236.98 mg | Cholesterol: 83.31 mg

Chicken Paillards with Mushrooms

Cremini mushrooms are baby portobellos. They are a creamy color, with brown caps.

INGREDIENTS | SERVES 4

4 (3-ounce) chicken breasts

3 tablespoons flour

⅛ teaspoon salt

⅛ teaspoon cayenne pepper

½ teaspoon dried marjoram leaves

2 tablespoons olive oil

4 shallots, minced

1 cup sliced button mushrooms

1 cup sliced cremini mushrooms

½ cup Low-Sodium Chicken Broth (see Chapter 13)

¼ cup dry white wine

1 teaspoon Worcestershire sauce

1 tablespoon cornstarch

Paillard

Paillard is a French word that literally means "bawdy." In cooking, it means to pound chicken, veal, or beef to ¼" thickness, to tenderize the meat and make it cook very quickly. To pound, place the meat between 2 sheets of waxed paper and pound with a meat mallet, starting from the center of the meat, to desired thickness.

1. Place chicken breasts between 2 sheets of waxed paper; pound until ¼" thick.

2. On a shallow plate, combine flour, salt, pepper, and marjoram. Dredge chicken in flour mixture to coat.

3. In a large skillet, heat olive oil over medium heat. Add chicken; sauté on first side for 3 minutes, then carefully turn and cook for 1 minute longer. Remove to platter and cover to keep warm.

4. Add shallots and mushrooms to skillet; cook and stir for 4–5 minutes, until tender.

5. In a small bowl, combine broth, wine, Worcestershire sauce, and cornstarch; mix well. Add to mushroom mixture; bring to a boil.

6. Return chicken to skillet; cook until chicken is hot and sauce bubbles and thickens. Serve immediately over brown rice, couscous, or pasta.

♥ **PER SERVING** Calories: 270.13 | Fat: 8.25 g | Saturated fat: 1.71 g | Sodium: 167.63 mg | Cholesterol: 79.63 mg

Turkey Cutlets Parmesan

This classic dish is usually smothered in cheese, with deep-fried breaded turkey. This lighter version is just as delicious.

INGREDIENTS | SERVES 6

1 egg white

¼ cup dry bread crumbs

⅛ teaspoon pepper

4 tablespoons grated Parmesan cheese, divided

6 (4-ounce) turkey cutlets

2 tablespoons olive oil

1 (15-ounce) can no-salt tomato sauce

1 teaspoon dried Italian seasoning

½ cup finely shredded part-skim mozzarella cheese

1. Preheat the oven to 350°F. Spray a 2-quart baking dish with nonstick cooking spray and set aside.

2. In a shallow bowl, beat egg white until foamy.

3. On a plate, combine bread crumbs, pepper, and 2 tablespoons Parmesan. Dip the turkey cutlets into the egg white, then into the breadcrumb mixture, turning to coat.

4. In a large saucepan, heat olive oil over medium heat. Add cutlets; brown on both sides, about 2–3 minutes per side. Place in prepared baking dish.

5. Add tomato sauce and Italian seasoning to saucepan; bring to a boil.

6. Pour sauce over cutlets in baking pan; top with mozzarella cheese and remaining 2 tablespoons Parmesan. Bake for 25–35 minutes, or until sauce bubbles and cheese melts and begins to brown. Serve with pasta, if desired.

♥ **PER SERVING** Calories: 275.49 | Fat: 10.98 g | Saturated fat: 3.43 g | Sodium: 229.86 mg | Cholesterol: 88.13 mg

Turkey Breast with Dried Fruit

This is a good choice for smaller families celebrating Thanksgiving. The sauce is delicious over mashed potatoes or steamed brown rice.

INGREDIENTS | SERVES 6

1½ pounds bone-in turkey breast
⅛ teaspoon salt
⅛ teaspoon pepper
1 tablespoon flour
1 tablespoon olive oil
1 tablespoon butter or plant sterol margarine
½ cup chopped prunes
½ cup chopped dried apricots
2 Granny Smith apples, peeled and chopped
1 cup Low-Sodium Chicken Broth (see Chapter 13)
¼ cup Madeira wine

1. Sprinkle turkey with salt, pepper, and flour.

2. In a large saucepan, heat olive oil and margarine over medium heat. Add turkey and cook until browned, about 5 minutes. Turn turkey.

3. Add all fruit to saucepan along with broth and wine.

4. Cover and bring to a simmer. Reduce heat to medium-low and simmer for 55–65 minutes, or until turkey is thoroughly cooked. Serve with fruit and sauce.

♥ **PER SERVING** Calories: 293.15 | Fat: 6.01 g | Saturated fat: 1.94 g | Sodium: 127.28 mg | Cholesterol: 78.37 mg

Turkey Curry with Fruit

This simple dish is fancy enough for company. Serve it with a brown rice pilaf and some toasted whole wheat French bread.

INGREDIENTS | SERVES 6

6 (4-ounce) turkey cutlets
1 tablespoon flour
1 tablespoon plus 1 teaspoon curry powder, divided
1 tablespoon olive oil
2 pears, chopped
1 apple, chopped
½ cup raisins
1 tablespoon sugar
⅛ teaspoon salt
⅓ cup apricot jam

1. Preheat the oven to 350°F. Spray a cookie sheet sides with nonstick cooking spray. Arrange cutlets on prepared cookie sheet.

2. In a small bowl, combine flour, 1 tablespoon curry powder, and olive oil; mix well. Spread evenly over cutlets.

3. In a medium bowl, combine pears, apple, raisins, sugar, salt, 1 teaspoon curry powder, and apricot jam; mix well. Divide this mixture over the cutlets.

4. Bake for 35–45 minutes. Serve immediately.

♥ **PER SERVING** Calories: 371.52 | Fat: 11.15 g | Saturated fat: 2.80 g | Sodium: 121.35 mg | Cholesterol: 78.24 mg

Chicken Pesto

*Pesto can be made with any nut. Hazelnuts are especially good at lowering
LDL cholesterol, and they're delicious in this green sauce.*

INGREDIENTS | SERVES 6

1 cup packed fresh basil leaves

¼ cup toasted chopped hazelnuts

2 cloves garlic, chopped

2 tablespoons olive oil

1 tablespoon water

¼ cup grated Parmesan cheese

½ cup Low-Sodium Chicken Broth (see Chapter 13)

12 ounces boneless, skinless chicken breasts

1 (12-ounce) package angel hair pasta

Herbs

Fresh herbs should be part of a healthy diet, simply because their wonderful tastes and aromas will let you reduce salt and fat without feeling deprived. Fresh herbs like basil, thyme, and oregano are also easy to grow in a pot on your windowsill. You can substitute dried herbs for fresh in a 3:1 ratio. For every tablespoon of fresh, use a teaspoon of dried.

1. Bring a large pot of salted water to a boil.

2. In a blender or food processor, combine basil, hazelnuts, and garlic; blend or process until very finely chopped. Add olive oil and water; blend until a paste forms. Then blend in Parmesan cheese; set aside.

3. In a large skillet, bring broth to a simmer over medium heat. Cut chicken into strips; add to broth. Cook for 4 minutes, then add the pasta to the boiling water.

4. Cook pasta for 1–2 minutes according to package directions, until al dente. Drain and add to chicken mixture; cook and stir for 1 minute until chicken is thoroughly cooked.

5. Add basil mixture; remove from heat and stir until a sauce forms. Serve immediately.

♥ **PER SERVING** Calories: 373.68 | Fat: 11.06 g | Saturated fat: 2.01 g | Sodium: 108.92 mg | Cholesterol: 38.04 mg

Cold Chicken with Cherry Tomato Sauce

*This is nice for a hot summer day. Prepare the chicken early in the day,
then quickly make the sauce, slice the chicken, and serve.*

INGREDIENTS | SERVES 3

2 teaspoons fresh thyme leaves

½ cup Low-Sodium Chicken Broth (see Chapter 13)

12 ounces boneless, skinless chicken breasts

1 tablespoon olive oil

3 cloves garlic, minced

2 cups cherry tomatoes

½ cup no-salt tomato juice

½ cup chopped fresh basil

¼ cup low-fat sour cream

⅛ teaspoon white pepper

1. In a large saucepan, combine thyme and chicken broth; bring to a simmer over medium heat.

2. Add chicken; reduce heat to low. Cover and poach for 7–9 minutes, or until chicken is thoroughly cooked.

3. Place chicken in a casserole dish just large enough to hold chicken. Pour poaching liquid over; cover and refrigerate at least 8 hours.

4. When ready to eat, heat olive oil in large skillet. Add garlic; cook and stir for 1 minute. Stir in tomatoes; cook and stir until the tomatoes pop, about 4–6 minutes. Add tomato juice, basil, sour cream, and pepper; stir, and heat briefly.

5. Slice the chicken and fan out on serving plate. Top with tomato mixture, and serve immediately.

♥ **PER SERVING** Calories: 227.58 | Fat: 8.63 g | Saturated fat: 2.57 g | Sodium: 198.32 mg | Cholesterol: 73.64 mg

Spicy Rib Eye in Red Sauce

This is one way to stretch a steak to serve six people. It's full of flavor, and easy, too.

INGREDIENTS | SERVES 6

1¼ pounds rib eye steak

⅛ teaspoon salt

⅛ teaspoon cayenne pepper

1 tablespoon olive oil

1 onion, chopped

3 cloves garlic, minced

⅓ cup dry red wine

1 tablespoon chili powder

½ teaspoon crushed red pepper flakes

½ teaspoon coriander seed

1 (20-ounce) can no-salt crushed tomatoes

1. Trim excess fat from steak; sprinkle with salt and pepper.

2. Heat a skillet over medium-high heat; add olive oil. Add steak; cook without moving until steak is browned, about 4–6 minutes. Turn and cook 2–3 minutes on second side, until medium-rare. Remove to plate.

3. Add onion and garlic to drippings remaining in skillet. Cook and stir until tender, about 4 minutes.

4. Add wine, chili powder, red pepper, coriander, and tomatoes; bring to a simmer. Reduce heat to low and simmer 15 minutes, until sauce is reduced and thickened.

5. Thinly slice steak against the grain; add to the sauce. Cook and stir 2–3 minutes, or until steak is hot and tender and sauce is blended. Serve immediately over brown rice, couscous, quinoa, or pasta.

♥ **PER SERVING** Calories: 267.81 | Fat: 10.22 g | Saturated fat: 3.27 g | Sodium: 138.71 mg | Cholesterol: 77.35 mg

Sirloin Meatballs in Sauce

Cooking meatballs in a sauce keeps them moist and tender. Serve this with hot cooked pasta or brown rice.

INGREDIENTS | SERVES 6; SERVING SIZE 2 MEATBALLS

1 tablespoon olive oil

3 cloves garlic, minced

½ cup minced onion

2 egg whites

½ cup dry bread crumbs

¼ cup grated Parmesan cheese

½ teaspoon crushed fennel seeds

½ teaspoon dried oregano leaves

2 teaspoons Worcestershire sauce

⅛ teaspoon pepper

⅛ teaspoon crushed red pepper flakes

1 pound (95% lean) ground sirloin

1 recipe Low-Fat Tomato Sauce (see Chapter 15)

Freezing Meatballs

Place meatballs on a cookie sheet. Bake at 375°F for 15–25 minutes, or until meatballs are browned and cooked through. Cool for 30 minutes, then chill until cold. Freeze individually, then pack into freezer bags. To thaw, let stand in refrigerator overnight.

1. In a small saucepan, heat olive oil over medium heat. Add garlic and onion; cook and stir until tender, about 5 minutes. Remove from heat and place in large mixing bowl.

2. Add egg whites, bread crumbs, Parmesan, fennel, oregano, Worcestershire sauce, pepper, and pepper flakes; mix well.

3. Add sirloin; mix gently but thoroughly until combined. Form into 12 meatballs.

4. In a large nonstick saucepan, place Spaghetti Sauce; bring to a simmer. Carefully add meatballs; return to a simmer, partially cover, and simmer 15–25 minutes, or until meatballs are thoroughly cooked.

♥ **PER SERVING** Calories: 367.93 | Fat: 13.56 g | Saturated fat: 3.91 g | Sodium: 305.47 mg | Cholesterol: 61.12 mg

Steak with Mushroom Sauce

A rich mushroom sauce adds great flavor to tender marinated steak. This is a recipe for company!

INGREDIENTS | SERVES 6

1–1¼ pounds flank steak

2 tablespoons red wine

1 tablespoon olive oil

1 tablespoon butter

1 onion, minced

1 (8-ounce) package sliced mushrooms

2 tablespoons flour

1½ cups Low-Sodium Beef Broth (see Chapter 13)

¼ teaspoon ground coriander

2 teaspoons Worcestershire sauce

⅛ teaspoon pepper

1. In a glass dish, combine steak, wine, and olive oil. Cover and marinate at least 8 hours.

2. When ready to eat, prepare and preheat grill. Drain steak, reserving marinade.

3. In a large skillet, melt butter over medium heat. Add onion and mushrooms; cook and stir until liquid evaporates, about 8–9 minutes.

4. Stir in flour; cook and stir for 2 minutes. Add beef broth and marinade from beef; bring to a boil. Stir in coriander, Worcestershire, and pepper; reduce heat to low and simmer while cooking steak.

5. Cook steak 6" from medium coals for 7–10 minutes, turning once, until steak reaches desired doneness. Remove from heat, cover, and let stand for 10 minutes.

6. Slice thinly against the grain, and serve with mushroom sauce.

♥ **PER SERVING** Calories: 262.45 | Fat: 16.09 g | Saturated fat: 6.42 g | Sodium: 114.22 mg | Cholesterol: 53.86 mg

Asian Beef Kabobs

Make sure that the wasabi powder is completely mixed with the olive oil before proceeding with the recipe, so the strong taste is evenly distributed.

INGREDIENTS | SERVES 4

2 tablespoons olive oil

1 teaspoon wasabi powder

1 tablespoon low-sodium soy sauce

1 tablespoon lemon juice

2 red bell peppers, sliced

1 (8-ounce) package cremini mushrooms

1 zucchini, sliced ½" thick

1 pound beef sirloin steak, cubed

Cremini Mushrooms

Cremini mushrooms are baby portobellos. These light-brown fungi have more flavor than button mushrooms. Because mushrooms don't synthesize sugars, they are very low in carbohydrates. They are a good source of fiber and niacin. They are fat free and cholesterol free and have a nice amount of fiber per serving.

1. In a small bowl, combine olive oil and wasabi powder; mix well. Add soy sauce and lemon juice; mix well.

2. Thread peppers, mushrooms, zucchini, and steak on metal skewers. Brush with the marinade; let stand for 10 minutes.

3. Prepare and preheat grill. Grill skewers 6" from medium coals for 7–10 minutes, turning once and brushing with wasabi mixture several times, until beef is desired doneness and vegetables are crisp-tender.

4. Serve immediately. Discard any remaining marinade.

♥ **PER SERVING** Calories: 254.80 | Fat: 9.55 g | Saturated fat: 2.76 g | Sodium: 217.78 mg | Cholesterol: 81.36 mg

Steak-and-Pepper Kabobs

Serve these kabobs with rice pilaf and a mixed fruit salad.

INGREDIENTS | SERVES 4

2 tablespoons brown sugar
½ teaspoon garlic powder
⅛ teaspoon cayenne pepper
¼ teaspoon onion salt
½ teaspoon chili powder
⅛ teaspoon ground cloves
1 (1-pound) sirloin steak, cut in 1" cubes
2 red bell peppers, cut in strips
2 green bell peppers, cut in strips

1. In a small bowl, combine brown sugar, garlic powder, cayenne, onion salt, chili powder, and clove; mix well.

2. Toss steak with brown sugar mixture. Place in glass dish and cover; refrigerate for 2 hours.

3. When ready to cook, prepare and preheat grill.

4. Thread steak cubes and pepper strips on metal skewers. Grill 6" from medium coals for 5–8 minutes, turning once, until steak is desired doneness and peppers are crisp-tender. Serve immediately.

♥ **PER SERVING** Calories: 205.53 | Fat: 6.23 g | Saturated fat: 2.24 g | Sodium: 133.03 mg | Cholesterol: 58.54 mg

Flank Steak with Mango Salsa

Meat and fruit is a wonderful combination; the sweetness of the fruit complements the tender richness of the meat. You can find mango salsa in your local grocery store.

INGREDIENTS | SERVES 4

2 mangoes, peeled
½ cup minced red onion
1 tablespoon grated fresh gingerroot
2 tablespoons lime juice
⅛ teaspoon salt
2 tablespoons honey
2 jalapeño peppers, minced
1 pound flank steak
¼ cup dry red wine
2 tablespoons olive oil
Mango salsa, to taste

1. Chop mangoes; combine in a small bowl with onion, gingerroot, lime juice, salt, honey, and jalapeño peppers. Stir, cover, and refrigerate while steak marinates.

2. Pierce steak with fork; combine in a glass dish with red wine and olive oil. Cover and marinate for 6–8 hours.

3. Preheat grill. Remove steak from marinade. Grill for 5–7 minutes on each side turning once.

4. Let steak stand, covered with foil, for 10 minutes; slice very thinly across the grain. Serve with mango salsa.

♥ **PER SERVING** Calories: 352.36 | Fat: 13.71 g | Saturated fat: 4.37 g | Sodium: 151.61 mg | Cholesterol: 58.51 mg

Whole-Grain Meatloaf

Here's a healthier take on the traditional meatloaf your grandmother used to make. Serve it with a big green salad or steamed vegetables.

INGREDIENTS | SERVES 8

1 tablespoon olive oil

1 onion, finely chopped

3 cloves garlic, minced

1 cup minced mushrooms

⅛ teaspoon pepper

1 teaspoon dried marjoram leaves

1 egg

1 egg white

½ cup chili sauce

¼ cup milk

1 tablespoon Worcestershire sauce

6 slices Whole-Grain Oatmeal Bread (see Chapter 16)

8 ounces (85% lean) ground beef

8 ounces ground turkey

8 ounces ground pork

3 tablespoons ketchup

Meatloaf Secrets

There are a few tricks to making the best meatloaf. First, combine all the other ingredients and mix well, then add the meat last. The less the meat is handled, the more tender the meatloaf will be. Then, when it's done baking, remove from the oven, cover with foil, and let sit for 10 minutes to let the juices redistribute.

1. Preheat oven to 325°F. Spray a 9" × 5" loaf pan with nonstick cooking spray and set aside.

2. In a large saucepan, heat olive oil over medium heat. Add onion, garlic, and mushrooms; cook and stir until tender, about 6 minutes. Place in large mixing bowl, sprinkle with pepper and marjoram; let stand for 15 minutes.

3. Add egg, egg white, chili sauce, milk, and Worcestershire sauce; mix well. Make crumbs from the oatmeal bread; add to onion mixture.

4. Add all of the meat; work gently with your hands just until combined. Press into prepared loaf pan. Top with ketchup. Bake for 60–75 minutes, or until internal temperature registers 165°F.

5. Remove from oven, cover with foil, and let stand for 10 minutes before slicing.

♥ **PER SERVING** Calories: 325.29 | Fat: 15.51 g | Saturated fat: 4.70 g | Sodium: 184.45 mg | Cholesterol: 90.46 mg

Filet Mignon with Vegetables

This is a wonderful dish for entertaining. The roasted vegetables are tender and sweet, and the meat is juicy.

INGREDIENTS | SERVES 8–10

1 (16-ounce) package baby carrots, halved lengthwise

1 (8-ounce) package frozen pearl onions

16 new potatoes, halved

2 tablespoons olive oil

2 pounds filet mignon

⅛ teaspoon salt

⅛ teaspoon white pepper

½ cup dry red wine

1. Preheat oven to 425°F.

2. Place carrots, onions, and potatoes in a large roasting pan. Drizzle with olive oil; toss to coat. Spread in an even layer. Roast for 15 minutes, then remove from oven.

3. Top with filet mignon; sprinkle meat with salt and pepper. Pour wine over meat and vegetables. Roast for 20–30 minutes longer, until beef registers 150°F for medium.

4. Remove from oven, tent with foil, and let stand for 5 minutes; carve to serve.

♥ **PER SERVING** Calories: 442.64 | Fat: 11.83 g | Saturated fat: 3.77 g | Sodium: 140.70 mg | Cholesterol: 70.55 mg

Corned Beef Hash

Serve this delicious hash on toasted Three-Grain French Bread (see Chapter 16), topped with scrambled eggs made with egg substitute.

INGREDIENTS | SERVES 6

2 tablespoons olive oil

2 onions, chopped

4 cloves garlic, minced

8 fingerling potatoes, chopped

4 carrots, chopped

¼ cup water

½ pound deli corned beef, diced

⅛ teaspoon ground cloves

⅛ teaspoon white pepper

3 tablespoons low-sodium chili sauce

1. Place olive oil in a large saucepan; heat over medium heat. Add onion and garlic; cook and stir for 3 minutes.

2. Add potatoes and carrots; cook and stir until potatoes are partially cooked, about 5 minutes.

3. Add water, corned beef, cloves, pepper, and chili sauce; stir well. Cover, reduce heat to low, and simmer for 10–15 minutes, or until blended and potatoes are cooked. Serve immediately.

♥ **PER SERVING** Calories: 283.21 | Fat: 11.97 g | Saturated fat: 3.09 g | Sodium: 472.63 mg | Cholesterol: 37.02 mg

Beef Risotto

This elegant recipe is perfect for a spring dinner. It is a last-minute recipe, so don't start it until after your guests have arrived.

INGREDIENTS | SERVES 6

2 cups water

2 cups Low-Sodium Beef Broth (see Chapter 13)

2 tablespoons olive oil

½ pound sirloin steak, chopped

1 onion, minced

2 cloves garlic, minced

1½ cups arborio rice

2 tablespoons steak sauce

¼ teaspoon pepper

1 pound asparagus, cut into 2" pieces

¼ cup grated Parmesan cheese

1 tablespoon butter

1. In a medium saucepan, combine water and broth; heat over low heat until warm; keep on heat.

2. In a large saucepan, heat olive oil over medium heat. Add beef; cook and stir until browned. Remove from pan with slotted spoon and set aside.

3. Add onion and garlic to pan; cook and stir until crisp-tender, about 4 minutes.

4. Add rice; cook and stir for 2 minutes. Add the broth mixture, a cup at a time, stirring until the liquid is absorbed, about 15 minutes.

5. When there is 1 cup broth remaining, return the beef to the pot; add steak sauce, pepper, and asparagus.

6. Cook and stir until rice is tender, beef is cooked, and asparagus is tender, about 5 minutes. Stir in Parmesan and butter, and serve immediately.

♥ **PER SERVING** Calories: 365.04 | Fat: 11.67 g | Saturated fat: 4.09 g | Sodium: 138.81 mg | Cholesterol: 36.20 mg

Beef with Mushroom Kabobs

Serve these kabobs with cooked brown rice and a tomato and spinach salad.

INGREDIENTS | SERVES 4

¼ cup dry red wine

1 tablespoon olive oil

⅛ teaspoon salt

⅛ teaspoon cayenne pepper

1 tablespoon dried basil leaves

2 cloves garlic, minced

1 pound beef sirloin steak

½ pound button mushrooms

½ pound cremini mushrooms

1 tablespoon lemon juice

1. In a medium glass bowl, combine wine, olive oil, salt, pepper, basil leaves, and garlic; mix well.

2. Cut steak into 1½" cubes; add to wine mixture. Stir to coat; cover and refrigerate for 1 hour.

3. Prepare and preheat grill. Drain steak, reserving marinade.

4. Trim mushroom stems and discard; brush mushrooms with lemon juice. Thread steak and mushrooms onto metal skewers.

5. Grill for 7–10 minutes, turning once and brushing with marinade, until beef is deep golden-brown and mushrooms are tender. Discard remaining marinade.

♥ **PER SERVING** Calories: 215.70 | Fat: 7.08 g | Saturated fat: 2.39 g | Sodium: 101.33 mg | Cholesterol: 78.63 mg

Barbecue Pork Chops

You can make lots of this excellent barbecue sauce and freeze it in 1-cup portions to use throughout the summer on everything from ribs to chicken.

INGREDIENTS | SERVES 8

2 tablespoons olive oil

1 onion, chopped

4 cloves garlic, minced

1 (14-ounce) can no-salt crushed tomatoes, undrained

1 cup low-sodium chili sauce

1 tablespoon lemon juice

2 tablespoons mustard

¼ cup brown sugar

2 tablespoons molasses

½ teaspoon cumin

1 teaspoon dried thyme leaves

⅛ teaspoon ground cloves

8 (3-ounce) boneless pork chops

Barbecue Sauce on the Grill

Most barbecue sauces should be added to the meat during the last part of grilling time. Since these sauces are usually high in sugar, they can burn easily on the high heat of the grill. Brush sauces onto the meat when they are almost fully cooked. The purpose of the sauce is to provide a glaze and add a layer of flavor.

1. In a large pot, heat olive oil over medium heat. Add onion and garlic; cook and stir for 3–4 minutes, until crisp-tender.

2. Add tomatoes, chili sauce, lemon juice, mustard, sugar, molasses, cumin, thyme, and cloves. Bring to a simmer; reduce heat, cover, and simmer for 2 hours.

3. When ready to cook, prepare and preheat grill. Spray grill rack with nonstick cooking spray and add pork chops.

4. Grill until the chops can be easily moved, about 4 minutes. Turn and brush with sauce. Cook for 3–5 minutes longer, or until chops are just pink, turning again and brushing with more sauce. Serve with sauce that hasn't been used to brush the pork.

♥ **PER SERVING** Calories: 276.23 | Fat: 11.80 g | Saturated fat: 3.53 g | Sodium: 417.98 mg | Cholesterol: 43.68 mg

Pork Chops with Cabbage

Cabbage is the ideal accompaniment to pork. It's tangy and sweet and becomes very tender when cooked in the slow cooker.

INGREDIENTS | SERVES 6

1 red onion, chopped
4 cloves garlic, minced
3 cups chopped red cabbage
3 cups chopped green cabbage
1 apple, chopped
6 (3-ounce) boneless pork chops
⅛ teaspoon white pepper
1 tablespoon olive oil
¼ cup brown sugar
¼ cup apple cider vinegar
1 tablespoon mustard

1. In a 4–5-quart slow cooker, combine onion, garlic, cabbages, and apple; mix well.

2. Trim pork chops of any excess fat; sprinkle with pepper. Heat olive oil in a large saucepan over medium heat. Brown chops on just one side, about 3 minutes. Add to slow cooker with vegetables.

3. In a small bowl, combine brown sugar, vinegar, and mustard; mix well. Pour into slow cooker. Cover and cook on low for 7–8 hours, or until pork and cabbage are tender. Serve immediately.

♥ **PER SERVING** Calories: 242.86 | Fat: 10.57 g | Saturated fat: 3.37 g | Sodium: 364.80 mg | Cholesterol: 43.68 mg

Mustard Pork Tenderloin

Mustard and low-fat sour cream coat the pork tenderloin to keep in moisture while it slowly roasts to perfection.

INGREDIENTS | SERVES 6

2 tablespoons red wine
1 tablespoon sugar
1 tablespoon olive oil
1¼ pounds pork tenderloin
¼ cup low-fat sour cream
3 tablespoons Dijon mustard
1 tablespoon minced fresh chives

1. In a glass baking dish, combine red wine, sugar, and olive oil. Add pork tenderloin; turn to coat. Cover and refrigerate for 8 hours.

2. Let pork stand at room temperature for 20 minutes. Preheat oven to 325°F. Roast for 30 minutes, basting occasionally with the marinade.

3. In a small bowl, combine sour cream, mustard, and chives; spread over tenderloin. Continue roasting 25–35 minutes, or until pork registers 160°F. Let stand for 5 minutes, then slice to serve.

♥ **PER SERVING** Calories: 209.84 | Fat: 9.08 g | Saturated fat: 2.98 g | Sodium: 147.13 mg | Cholesterol: 83.83 mg

Canadian Bacon Risotto

Risotto has a reputation for being difficult to make, but it's not.
Just add the warm broth gradually and keep stirring!

INGREDIENTS | **SERVES 6**

2 cups water

3 cups Low-Sodium Chicken Broth (see Chapter 13)

1 tablespoon olive oil

1 chopped onion

3 cloves garlic, minced

1 (8-ounce) package sliced mushrooms

½ teaspoon dried oregano leaves

1 teaspoon dried basil leaves

2 cups arborio rice

⅛ teaspoon white pepper

1 cup chopped Canadian bacon

¼ cup shredded Parmesan cheese

1 tablespoon butter

1. In a medium saucepan, combine water and broth; heat over low heat until warm; keep on heat.

2. In a large saucepan, heat olive oil over medium heat. Add onion, garlic, and mushrooms; cook and stir until crisp-tender, about 4 minutes. Add oregano and basil.

3. Add rice; cook and stir 2 minutes. Add broth mixture, a cup at a time, stirring until the liquid is absorbed, about 15 minutes.

4. When there is 1 cup broth remaining, add pepper and Canadian bacon along with the last cup of broth. Cook and stir until rice is tender, about 5 minutes.

5. Stir in Parmesan and butter, and serve immediately.

♥ **PER SERVING** Calories: 379.72 | Fat: 9.41 g | Saturated fat: 3.17 g | Sodium: 292.55 mg | Cholesterol: 26.94 mg

Canadian Bacon

In the United States, Canadian bacon is simply lean bacon, or smoked back bacon. But in Canada, it's a specific cut of ham called Canadian peameal. It's a lean cut of cured pork. It used to be rolled in ground yellow peas, which extended the shelf life; now it's rolled in ground corn. You can order the real Canadian peameal bacon online.

Western Omelet

This classic omelet can be made with a jalapeño or habanero pepper thrown in if you like it really spicy.

INGREDIENTS | SERVES 4

1 tablespoon olive oil
½ cup chopped onion
3 cloves garlic, minced
½ cup chopped green bell pepper
½ cup chopped red bell pepper
3 ounces chopped ham
1 egg
8 egg whites
¼ teaspoon cayenne pepper
1 teaspoon chili powder
¼ cup skim milk
⅛ teaspoon pepper

1. In a large nonstick skillet, heat olive oil over medium heat. Add onion, garlic, and bell peppers; cook and stir until crisp-tender, about 4 minutes. Add ham; cook and stir until ham is hot.

2. In a large bowl, combine egg, egg whites, cayenne pepper, chili powder, milk, and pepper; mix well. Pour into skillet with vegetables and ham.

3. Cook, running a spatula around the edges to let uncooked mixture flow underneath, until eggs are set and bottom is golden brown. Fold omelet over, and serve.

♥ **PER SERVING** Calories: 216.81 | Fat: 13.12 g | Saturated fat: 5.15 g | Sodium: 477.02 mg | Cholesterol: 81.19 mg

Pork Scallops Françoise

This fresh and simple recipe takes just minutes to make. Use the best ingredients you can find for the perfect meal.

INGREDIENTS | SERVES 4

3 tablespoons flour
⅛ teaspoon salt
⅛ teaspoon pepper
1 egg white, slightly beaten
4 (3-ounce) pork scallops
1 tablespoon olive oil
1 tablespoon butter
3 cloves garlic, minced
2 tablespoons lemon juice
2 tablespoons chopped fresh parsley

1. On a plate, combine flour, salt, and pepper. Place egg white in a shallow bowl.

2. If necessary, pound scallops until they are ⅛" thick. Dip scallops into flour, then into egg white mixture.

3. Heat olive oil and butter in a nonstick skillet. Add garlic; cook for 1 minute. Add coated pork; brown for 2–3 minutes per side.

4. Add lemon juice; cook for 2–3 minute. Sprinkle with parsley, and serve immediately.

♥ **PER SERVING** Calories: 224.74 | Fat: 11.25 g | Saturated fat: 4.04 g | Sodium: 158.05 mg | Cholesterol: 80.87 mg

Pork Scallops with Spinach

A simple creamed spinach tops tender pork scallops in this easy recipe for dinner.

INGREDIENTS | SERVES 6

3 tablespoons flour

⅛ teaspoon salt

⅛ teaspoon pepper

6 (3-ounce) pork scallops

2 tablespoons olive oil

1 onion, chopped

1 (10-ounce) package frozen chopped spinach, thawed

1 tablespoon flour

½ teaspoon celery seed

⅓ cup nonfat light cream

⅓ cup part-skim ricotta cheese

½ cup dried bread crumbs, divided

2 tablespoons grated Romano cheese

1. Preheat the oven to 350°F.

2. On a plate, combine 3 tablespoons flour, salt, and pepper; mix well. Pound pork scallops, if necessary, to ⅛" thickness.

3. Heat olive oil in a nonstick pan over medium high heat. Dredge pork in flour mixture and sauté in pan, turning once, until just browned, about 1 minute per side. Remove to a baking dish.

4. Add onion to pan; cook and stir for 3 minutes.

5. Drain spinach well and add to pan; cook and stir until liquid evaporates.

6. Add flour and celery seed; cook and stir for 1 minute.

7. Stir in light cream; cook and stir until thickened, about 3 minutes. Remove from heat and add ricotta cheese and half of the bread crumbs.

8. Divide spinach mixture on top of pork in baking dish. Top with remaining bread crumbs and Romano. Bake for 10–15 minutes, or until pork is tender and thoroughly cooked. Serve immediately.

♥ **PER SERVING** Calories: 298.66 | Fat: 12.60 g | Saturated fat: 4.08 g | Sodium: 303.25 mg | Cholesterol: 80.88 mg

Fruit-Stuffed Pork Tenderloin

Perfect for entertaining, you can make this recipe ahead of time. Stuff the pork mixture, then brown and bake it just before serving.

INGREDIENTS | SERVES 6

1½ pounds pork tenderloin

¼ cup dry white wine

6 prunes, chopped

5 dried apricots, chopped

1 onion, chopped

2 tablespoons flour

⅛ teaspoon salt

⅛ teaspoon pepper

2 tablespoons olive oil

½ cup Low-Sodium Chicken Broth (see Chapter 13)

1 teaspoon dried thyme leaves

1. Trim excess fat from meat. Cut lengthwise, cutting to but not through the other side. Open up the meat; place on work surface cut-side up. Lightly pound with a rolling pin or meat mallet until about ½" thick.

2. In a small saucepan, combine wine, prunes, apricots, and onion. Simmer for 10 minutes, or until fruit is soft and wine is absorbed. Place mixture in center of tenderloin. Roll pork around fruit mixture, using a toothpick to secure.

3. Sprinkle pork with flour, salt, and pepper.

4. In an ovenproof saucepan, heat olive oil. Add pork; brown on all sides, turning frequently, about 5–6 minutes.

5. Add broth and thyme; bake 25–35 minutes, or until internal temperature registers 155°F. Let stand 5 minutes; remove toothpicks, and slice to serve.

♥ **PER SERVING** Calories: 249.06 | Fat: 9.82 g | Saturated fat: 2.41 g | Sodium: 102.85 mg | Cholesterol: 72.51 mg

Risotto with Ham and Pineapple

This risotto is fresh and delicious, reminiscent of Hawaii! Serve it with a green salad and some sherbet for dessert.

INGREDIENTS | SERVES 4–6

2 cups water

2 cups Low-Sodium Chicken Broth (see Chapter 13)

1 tablespoon olive oil

1 tablespoon butter

1 onion, chopped

3 cloves garlic, minced

½ teaspoon dried thyme leaves

1 red bell pepper, chopped

1½ cups arborio rice

1 cup chopped ham

1 (20-ounce) can pineapple tidbits, drained

⅛ teaspoon pepper

¼ cup grated Parmesan cheese

1. In a medium saucepan, combine water and chicken broth; bring to a simmer over low heat. Keep warm.

2. In a large saucepan, heat olive oil and butter over medium heat. Add onion and garlic; cook and stir for 3 minutes.

3. Add thyme, bell pepper, and rice; cook and stir for 4 minutes.

4. Start adding the broth, 1 cup at a time, stirring frequently. When 1 cup broth remains to be added, add ham, pineapple, and pepper to risotto.

5. Add last cup of broth; cook and stir until rice is tender and creamy and liquid is absorbed. Stir in Parmesan; cover, let stand for 5 minutes, then serve.

♥ **PER SERVING** Calories: 369.77 | Fat: 8.92 g | Saturated fat: 3.17 g | Sodium: 390.26 mg | Cholesterol: 26.81 mg

Pork Skewers with Cherry Tomatoes

Cherry tomatoes, when grilled, burst with flavor in your mouth. Serve these kabobs with a rice pilaf.

INGREDIENTS | SERVES 4

¾ pound pork tenderloin, cubed

24 cherry tomatoes

1 onion, cut into eighths

2 tablespoons olive oil

1 tablespoon lemon juice

⅛ teaspoon pepper

2 tablespoons chopped flat-leaf parsley

1 tablespoon fresh oregano leaves

¼ cup shredded Parmesan cheese

Parmesan: Shredded or Grated?

There is quite a difference in the amounts when Parmesan cheese is shredded versus grated. Shredded cheese is in strips, and the total amount will be less. Grated is very finely shredded cheese, and you'll end up eating more of it. They both will give about the same flavor and taste. Be sure to read packages carefully if you buy cheese already shredded.

1. Prepare and preheat grill. Thread pork, cherry tomatoes, and onion on metal skewers.

2. In a small bowl, combine olive oil, lemon juice, pepper, parsley, and oregano; brush skewers with olive oil mixture.

3. Grill skewers 6" from medium coals for 8–10 minutes, turning and brushing occasionally with marinade, until pork registers 155°F.

4. Sprinkle with Parmesan; let stand to melt, and serve.

♥ **PER SERVING** Calories: 240.01 | Fat: 10.48 g | Saturated fat: 3.50 g | Sodium: 177.18 mg | Cholesterol: 78.34 mg

Herb-Crusted Pork Tenderloin

Pork tenderloin is a cut with very little fat; it is tender and delicious.

INGREDIENTS | SERVES 8

⅓ cup chopped flat-leaf parsley

4 fresh sage leaves, chopped

¼ cup dried bread crumbs

2 tablespoons fresh thyme leaves

1 tablespoon mustard

1 tablespoon olive oil

2 (1-pound) pork tenderloins

⅛ teaspoon salt

⅛ teaspoon pepper

2 tablespoons olive oil

1. Preheat the oven to 400°F.

2. On a shallow plate, combine parsley, sage, bread crumbs, and thyme; mix until combined. Add mustard and olive oil; toss until combined. Set aside.

3. Sprinkle tenderloins with salt and pepper.

4. Heat 2 tablespoons olive oil in a heavy ovenproof saucepan over medium-high heat. Sear tenderloins on all sides, about 2 minutes a side, until golden brown.

5. Remove pan from heat; carefully press herb mixture onto top and sides of tenderloins. Roast for 15–20 minutes, or until internal temperature registers 155°F.

6. Let stand for 5 minutes; serve.

♥ **PER SERVING** Calories: 199.58 | Fat: 9.77 g | Saturated fat: 2.63 g | Sodium: 139.95 mg | Cholesterol: 74.84 mg

Prosciutto Fruit Omelet

*Ham and fruit are a classic combination. You can peel the apple
or not, as you wish; unpeeled, it has more fiber.*

INGREDIENTS | SERVES 4

¼ pound thinly sliced prosciutto

½ cup shredded part-skim mozzarella cheese

2 tablespoons grated Parmesan cheese

1 egg

8 egg whites

¼ cup low-fat sour cream

⅛ teaspoon pepper

1 tablespoon olive oil

1 apple, chopped

Prosciutto

Prosciutto is an Italian ham that has been dry-cured and smoked. It's usually available at the deli counter and is very thinly sliced. The best prosciutto is cured for at least two years. This ham is usually very highly marbled. Even though purists would shudder, you can cut off the visible fat and discard it to reduce the fat content.

1. Trim off excess fat from prosciutto and discard. Thinly slice; combine with cheeses. Set aside.

2. In a large bowl, combine egg, egg whites, sour cream, and pepper; mix well.

3. In a large nonstick saucepan, heat olive oil over medium heat; add apples and cook and stir until apples are tender. Pour in egg mixture. Cook, running a spatula around the edges to let uncooked mixture flow underneath, until eggs are almost set and bottom is golden brown.

4. Sprinkle with cheese and ham mixture; cook for 2–3 minutes longer.

5. Cover, remove from heat, and let stand for 2 minutes. Fold omelet over on itself, slide onto serving plate, and serve.

♥ **PER SERVING** Calories: 221.48 | Fat: 12.35 g | Saturated fat: 4.99 g | Sodium: 551.41 mg | Cholesterol: 80.91 mg

Asian Pork Stir-Fry

Serve this delicious and spicy stir-fry over hot cooked brown rice, with chopsticks.

INGREDIENTS | **SERVES 6**

1 tablespoon low-sodium soy sauce

2 tablespoons honey

2 tablespoons water

½ teaspoon wasabi powder

1 tablespoon cornstarch

2 tablespoons canola oil

3 cloves garlic, minced

1 tablespoon minced gingerroot

1 pound pork tenderloin, sliced

1 red bell pepper, chopped

1 (8-ounce) package cremini mushrooms, sliced

2 zucchini, sliced

8 ounces snow peas

1. In a small bowl, combine soy sauce, honey, water, wasabi powder, and cornstarch; mix thoroughly with wire whisk. Set aside. Prepare the meat and all of the vegetables.

2. In a large wok or large skillet, heat canola oil over medium-high heat. Add garlic and ginger; stir-fry for 2 minutes.

3. Add pork tenderloin slices; stir-fry for 3–4 minutes. Remove pork from wok.

4. Add bell pepper, mushrooms, zucchini, and snow peas; stir-fry until crisp-tender, about 4 minutes.

5. Return meat to wok. Stir soy sauce mixture; pour into wok. Stir-fry for 2–4 minutes, or until sauce boils and thickens. Serve immediately.

♥ **PER SERVING** Calories: 214.75 | Fat: 9.01 g | Saturated fat: 1.81 g | Sodium: 147.48 mg | Cholesterol: 49.90 mg

CHAPTER 15

Heart-Healthy Fish, Pasta, and Bean Main-Dish Recipes

Seafood Risotto

Risotto is an elegant dish, perfect for entertaining. Do all your prep work ahead of time and store ingredients in the fridge, and the dish will only take about 30 minutes of cooking time.

INGREDIENTS | SERVES 6

2 cups water

2½ cups Low-Sodium Chicken Broth (see Chapter 13)

2 tablespoons olive oil

1 onion, minced

3 cloves garlic, minced

1½ cups arborio rice

1 cup chopped celery

1 tablespoon fresh dill weed

¼ cup dry white wine

½ pound sole fillets

¼ pound small raw shrimp

½ pound bay scallops

¼ cup grated Parmesan cheese

1 tablespoon butter

1. In a medium saucepan, combine water and broth; heat over low heat. Keep on heat.

2. In a large saucepan, heat olive oil over medium heat. Add onion and garlic; cook and stir until crisp-tender, about 3 minutes.

3. Add rice; cook and stir for 3 minutes.

4. Start adding broth mixture, a cup at a time, stirring frequently and adding liquid when previous addition is absorbed.

5. When only 1 cup of broth remains stir in celery, dill, wine, fish fillets, shrimp, and scallops; add last cup of broth.

6. Cook, stirring constantly, 5–7 minutes, or until fish is cooked and rice is tender and creamy. Stir in Parmesan and butter; serve.

♥ **PER SERVING** Calories: 397.22 | Fat: 11.11 g | Saturated fat: 3.20 g | Sodium: 354.58 mg | Cholesterol: 94.39 mg

Citrus-Blueberry Fish en Papillote

This gorgeous presentation of a healthy dish is worthy of company!
Serve it with brown rice pilaf and a baby spinach salad.

INGREDIENTS | SERVES 4

1 tablespoon olive oil
1 onion, finely chopped
4 cloves garlic, minced
2 tablespoons lemon juice
2 tablespoons orange juice
1 teaspoon orange zest
4 (4-ounce) sole or mahi mahi fillets
1 cup blueberries
2 tablespoons blueberry jam

En Papillote

This French term means "in parchment"; as a cooking term it means food cooked while completely sealed in parchment paper. This method keeps the food moist and prevents overcooking, while sealing in the flavors. You can also use heavy-duty aluminum foil instead of parchment paper.

1. Preheat the oven to 400°F. Cut parchment paper into 4 large heart shapes measuring about 12" × 18". Fold hearts in half, open up, then set aside.

2. In a small saucepan, heat olive oil over medium heat. Add onion and garlic; cook and stir for 4 minutes, until crisp-tender. Remove from heat and stir in lemon and orange juices and orange zest.

3. Place 1 fillet at the center of each parchment heart, next to the fold. Divide onion mixture among fillets.

4. In small bowl, combine blueberries and blueberry jam; mix gently. Divide on top of onion mixture.

5. Fold one half of the parchment heart over the other. Crimp and fold the edges to seal. Place on cookie sheets.

6. Bake for 18–23 minutes, or until the bundles are puffed and the paper is browned. Serve immediately, warning diners to be careful of the steam that will billow out when the packages are opened.

♥ **PER SERVING** Calories: 220.81 | Fat: 5.18 g | Saturated fat: 0.87 g | Sodium: 116.46 mg | Cholesterol: 72.25 mg

Cajun-Rubbed Fish

Fish should never be marinated longer than 1 hour; otherwise, the flesh may become mushy. This is a perfect last-minute dish for entertaining.

INGREDIENTS | SERVES 4

½ teaspoon black pepper
¼ teaspoon cayenne pepper
½ teaspoon lemon zest
½ teaspoon dried dill weed
⅛ teaspoon salt
1 tablespoon brown sugar
4 (5-ounce) swordfish steaks

1. Prepare and preheat grill.

2. In a small bowl, combine pepper, cayenne, lemon zest, dill weed, salt, and brown sugar; mix well. Sprinkle onto both sides of swordfish; rub in. Set aside for 30 minutes.

3. Brush grill with oil. Add swordfish; cook without moving for 4 minutes.

4. Carefully turn steaks and cook for 2–4 minutes on second side, until fish just flakes when tested with fork. Serve immediately.

♥ **PER SERVING** Calories: 233.57 | Fat: 7.31 g | Saturated fat: 2.00 g | Sodium: 237.08 mg | Cholesterol: 70.83 mg

Broiled Swordfish

This flavorful sauce and cooking method can be used with any fish.

INGREDIENTS | SERVES 4

1 tablespoon olive oil
2 tablespoons dry white wine
1 teaspoon lemon zest
¼ teaspoon salt
⅛ teaspoon white pepper
1 teaspoon dried dill weed
1¼ pounds swordfish steaks
4 tomato slices, ½" thick

1. Preheat broiler.

2. In a small bowl, combine oil, wine, zest, salt, pepper, and dill weed; whisk to blend.

3. Place steaks on broiler pan; brush with oil mixture. Broil 6" from heat for 4 minutes. Turn fish; brush with remaining oil mixture. Top with tomatoes.

4. Return to oven; broil 4–6 minutes, or until fish flakes when tested with fork.

♥ **PER SERVING** Calories: 210.97 | Fat: 9.10 g | Saturated fat: 2.03 g | Sodium: 273.91 mg | Cholesterol: 55.25 mg

Baked Halibut in Mustard Sauce

Combining bread crumbs with milk to form a sauce is a trick from Scandinavian cooks.

INGREDIENTS | SERVES 4

1 pound halibut fillet

Pinch salt

⅛ teaspoon white pepper

1 tablespoon lemon juice

2 tablespoons butter or margarine, melted

¼ cup skim milk

2 tablespoons Dijon mustard

1 slice Honey-Wheat Sesame Bread (see Chapter 16), crumbled

1. Preheat the oven to 400°F. Spray a 1-quart baking dish with nonstick cooking spray.

2. Cut fish into serving-size pieces; sprinkle with salt, pepper, and lemon juice.

3. In a small bowl, combine butter, milk, and mustard; whisk until blended. Stir in bread crumbs; pour over fish.

4. Bake 20–25 minutes, or until fish flakes when tested with fork and sauce is bubbling. Serve immediately.

♥ **PER SERVING** Calories: 219.84 | Fat: 9.38 g | Saturated fat: 4.30 g | Sodium: 244.95 mg | Cholesterol: 54.29 mg

Bluefish with Asian Seasonings

Bluefish has a light and delicate texture and flavor.

INGREDIENTS | SERVES 4

1¼ pounds bluefish fillets

1 tablespoon lime juice

2 teaspoons low-sodium soy sauce

2 teaspoons grated gingerroot

3 cloves garlic, minced

1 teaspoon sesame oil

1 teaspoon Thai chile paste

1 tablespoon orange juice

⅛ teaspoon white pepper

1. Preheat broiler. Place bluefish fillets on a broiler pan.

2. In a small bowl, combine all remaining ingredients, being very careful to make sure chile paste is evenly distributed.

3. Pour sauce over fillets; broil 6" from heat for 6–9 minutes, or until fish is opaque and flakes when tested with fork. Serve immediately.

♥ **PER SERVING** Calories: 193.98 | Fat: 7.17 g | Saturated fat: 1.46 g | Sodium: 181.39 mg | Cholesterol: 83.58 mg

Poached Fish with Tomatoes and Capers

White fish fillets include cod, haddock, and pollock. This mild and sweet fish cooks quickly.

INGREDIENTS | SERVES 4

2 tablespoons olive oil

½ cup chopped red onion

2 cloves garlic, minced

1 cup chopped fresh tomatoes

2 tablespoons no-salt tomato paste

¼ cup dry white wine

2 tablespoons capers, rinsed

4 (4-ounce) white fish fillets

¼ cup chopped parsley

1. In a large skillet, heat olive oil over medium heat. Add onion and garlic; cook and stir about 5 minutes.

2. Add tomatoes, tomato paste, and wine and bring to a simmer; simmer for 5 minutes, stirring frequently.

3. Add capers and stir; arrange fillets on top of sauce. Spoon sauce over fish.

4. Reduce heat to low; cover, and poach for 7–10 minutes, or until fish flakes when tested with fork. Sprinkle with parsley, and serve immediately.

♥ **PER SERVING** Calories: 191.05 | Fat: 7.70 g | Saturated fat: 1.13 g | Sodium: 199.73 mg | Cholesterol: 48.73 mg

Baked Lemon Sole with Herbed Crumbs

Adding herbs to bread crumbs is a wonderful way to make a flavorful crust on fish without adding calories, fat, or sodium.

INGREDIENTS | SERVES 4

2 slices Light Whole-Grain Bread (see Chapter 16), crumbled

2 tablespoons minced parsley

2 cloves garlic, minced

1 teaspoon dried dill weed

2 tablespoons olive oil

4 (6-ounce) sole fillets

2 tablespoons lemon juice

Pinch salt

⅛ teaspoon white pepper

1. Preheat the oven to 350°F.

2. In a small bowl, combine bread crumbs, parsley, garlic, and dill weed; mix well. Drizzle with olive oil; toss to coat.

3. Spray a 9" baking dish with nonstick cooking spray; arrange fillets in dish. Sprinkle with lemon juice, salt, and pepper. Divide crumb mixture on top of fillets.

4. Bake for 12–17 minutes, or until crumb topping is browned. Serve immediately.

♥ **PER SERVING** Calories: 294.58 | Fat: 9.86 g | Saturated fat: 1.65 g | Sodium: 288.21 mg | Cholesterol: 110.78 mg

Salmon with Mustard and Orange

*Mustard adds great flavor and helps cut the rich texture of salmon,
and orange adds a nice touch of sweetness.*

INGREDIENTS | SERVES 4

4 (5-ounce) salmon fillets
1 tablespoon olive oil
2 tablespoons Dijon mustard
1 tablespoon flour
1 teaspoon orange zest
2 tablespoons orange juice
Pinch salt
⅛ teaspoon white pepper

1. Preheat broiler. Place fillets on a broiler pan.

2. In a small bowl, combine remaining ingredients; mix well. Spread over salmon.

3. Broil fish 6" from heat for 7–10 minutes, or until fish flakes when tested with fork and topping bubbles and begins to brown. Serve immediately.

♥ **PER SERVING** Calories: 277.64 | Fat: 14.02 g | Saturated fat: 2.09 g | Sodium: 197.84 mg | Cholesterol: 90.53 mg

Red Snapper with Fruit Salsa

This colorful and healthy salsa is sweet and spicy, perfect with the roasted fish.

INGREDIENTS | SERVES 4

1 cup blueberries
1 cup chopped watermelon
1 jalapeño pepper, minced
½ cup chopped tomatoes
3 tablespoons olive oil, divided
2 tablespoons orange juice
⅛ teaspoon salt, divided
⅛ teaspoon white pepper
4 (4-ounce) red snapper fillets
1 lemon, thinly sliced

1. Preheat the oven to 400°F. Spray a 9" glass baking pan with nonstick cooking spray and set aside.

2. In a medium bowl, combine blueberries, watermelon, jalapeño pepper, tomatoes, 1 tablespoon olive oil, orange juice, and half of the salt; mix well and set aside.

3. Arrange fillets in prepared pan. Sprinkle with remaining salt and the white pepper; drizzle with 2 tablespoons olive oil. Top with lemon slices.

4. Bake for 15–20 minutes. Place on serving plate, and top with blueberry mixture; serve immediately.

♥ **PER SERVING** Calories: 254.40 | Fat: 12.01 g | Saturated fat: 1.82 g | Sodium: 186.42 mg | Cholesterol: 72.25 mg

Seared Scallops with Fruit

Serve this super quick and colorful dish with a brown rice pilaf and a green salad.

INGREDIENTS | SERVES 3–4

1 pound sea scallops

Pinch salt

⅛ teaspoon white pepper

1 tablespoon olive oil

1 tablespoon butter or margarine

2 peaches, sliced

¼ cup dry white wine

1 cup blueberries

1 tablespoon lime juice

Scallops

Scallops are a shellfish that is very low in fat. Sea scallops are the largest, followed by bay scallops and calico scallops. They should smell very fresh and slightly briny, like the sea. If they smell fishy, do not buy them. There may be a small muscle attached to the side of each scallop; pull that off and discard it, as it can be tough.

1. Rinse scallops; pat dry. Sprinkle with salt and pepper; set aside.

2. In a large skillet, heat olive oil and butter over medium-high heat. Add scallops; don't move them for 3 minutes. Carefully check to see if scallops are deep golden brown. If they are, turn and cook for 1–2 minutes on the second side; remove to serving plate.

3. Add peaches to skillet; brown quickly on one side, about 2 minutes. Turn peaches and add wine to skillet; bring to a boil.

4. Remove from heat and add blueberries; pour over scallops. Sprinkle with lime juice, and serve immediately.

♥ **PER SERVING** Calories: 207.89 | Fat: 7.36 g | Saturated fat: 2.40 g | Sodium: 242.16 mg | Cholesterol: 45.03 mg

Fennel-Grilled Haddock

Fennel is sweet and tastes like licorice, especially when grilled. It imparts its distinctive flavor to the mild fish using this grilling method.

INGREDIENTS | **SERVES 4**

2 bulbs fennel
4 (5-ounce) haddock or halibut steaks
3 tablespoons olive oil
Pinch salt
⅛ teaspoon cayenne pepper
1 teaspoon paprika
2 tablespoons lemon juice

1. Prepare and preheat grill.

2. Slice fennel bulbs lengthwise into ½" slices, leaving the stalks and fronds attached.

3. Brush fennel and haddock with olive oil on all sides to coat. Sprinkle fish with salt, pepper, and paprika.

4. Place fennel on grill 6" above medium coals, cut-side down. Arrange fish on top of fennel; close the grill.

5. Grill for 5–7 minutes, or until fennel is deep golden-brown and fish flakes when tested with fork.

6. Remove fish to serving platter; sprinkle with lemon juice, and cover.

7. Cut root end and stems from fennel and discard. Slice and place on top of fish; serve immediately.

♥ **PER SERVING** Calories: 246.68 | Fat: 11.35 g | Saturated fat: 1.58 g | Sodium: 192.31 mg | Cholesterol: 78.63 mg

Poached Chilean Sea Bass with Pears

Leave the skin on the pears for a pretty presentation and to keep the fruit from falling apart.

INGREDIENTS | SERVES 4

½ cup dry white wine

¼ cup water

2 bay leaves

⅛ teaspoon salt

½ teaspoon Tabasco sauce

1 lemon, thinly sliced

4 (4–5 ounce) sea bass steaks or fillets

2 firm pears, cored and cut in half

1 tablespoon butter

1. In a large skillet over medium heat, combine wine, water, bay leaves, salt, Tabasco, and lemon slices; bring to a simmer.

2. Add fish and pears. Reduce heat to low; poach 9–12 minutes, or until fish flakes when tested with a fork. Remove to serving platter.

3. Remove bay leaves from poaching liquid; increase heat to high. Boil for 3–5 minutes, or until liquid is reduced and syrupy. Swirl in butter; pour over fish and pears, and serve immediately.

♥ **PER SERVING** Calories: 235.38 | Fat: 5.81 g | Saturated fat: 2.55 g | Sodium: 194.06 mg | Cholesterol: 65.71 mg

Scallops on Skewers with Tomatoes

This sauce is originally from Argentina. It's fragrant and delicious.

INGREDIENTS | SERVES 4

1 pound sea scallops

12 cherry tomatoes

4 green onions, cut in half crosswise

½ cup chopped parsley

1 tablespoon fresh oregano leaves

3 tablespoons olive oil

2 tablespoons lemon juice

2 cloves garlic

⅛ teaspoon salt

⅛ teaspoon pepper

1. Prepare and preheat broiler. Rinse scallops and pat dry. Thread on skewers with cherry tomatoes and green onions.

2. In a blender or food processor, combine remaining ingredients; blend or process until smooth. Reserve ¼ cup of sauce.

3. Brush remaining sauce onto food on skewers. Place on broiler pan; broil 6" from heat for 3–4 minutes per side, turning once during cooking time. Serve with remaining sauce.

♥ **PER SERVING** Calories: 202.03 | Fat: 11.11 g | Saturated fat: 1.52 g | Sodium: 251.50 mg | Cholesterol: 35.06 mg

Almond Snapper with Shrimp Sauce

You could use any mild white fish in this delicious recipe.

INGREDIENTS | **SERVES 6**

1 egg white
¼ cup dry bread crumbs
⅓ cup ground almonds
⅛ teaspoon salt
⅛ teaspoon white pepper
6 (4-ounce) red snapper fillets
3 tablespoons olive oil, divided
1 onion, chopped
4 cloves garlic, minced
1 red bell pepper, chopped
¼ pound small raw shrimp
1 tablespoon lemon juice
½ cup low-fat sour cream
½ teaspoon dried dill weed

1. Place egg white in a shallow bowl; beat until foamy.

2. On a shallow plate, combine bread crumbs, almonds, salt, and pepper; mix well. Dip fish into egg white, then into crumb mixture, pressing to coat. Let stand on wire rack for 10 minutes.

3. In a small saucepan, heat 1 tablespoon olive oil over medium heat. Add onion, garlic, and bell pepper; cook and stir until tender, about 5 minutes.

4. Add shrimp; cook and stir just until shrimp curl and turn pink, about 1–2 minutes. Remove from heat and add lemon juice; set aside.

5. In a large saucepan, heat remaining 2 tablespoons olive oil over medium heat. Add coated fish fillets. Cook for 4 minutes on one side; carefully turn and cook for 2–5 minutes on second side, until coating is browned and fish flakes when tested with a fork.

6. While fish is cooking, return saucepan with shrimp to medium heat. Add sour cream and dill weed; heat, stirring, until mixture is hot.

7. Remove fish from skillet; place on serving plate. Top each with a spoonful of shrimp sauce, and serve immediately.

♥ **PER SERVING** Calories: 272.57 | Fat: 13.80 g | Saturated fat: 3.09 g | Sodium: 216.17 mg | Cholesterol: 88.71 mg

Scallops on Skewers with Lemon

Because scallops are so low in fat, sodium, and cholesterol, you can add a bit of low-sodium bacon to this dish for a flavor treat.

INGREDIENTS | SERVES 4

2 tablespoons lemon juice

1 teaspoon grated lemon zest

2 teaspoons sesame oil

2 tablespoons chili sauce

⅛ teaspoon cayenne pepper

1 pound sea scallops

4 strips low-sodium bacon

Bacon

If you read labels and choose carefully, bacon can be an occasional treat. Many companies now make low-sodium bacon. In health-food stores you can often find organic bacon that has better nutrition. Also consider Canadian bacon. More like ham, this meat has less sodium, fat, and chemicals like nitrates than regular bacon.

1. Prepare and preheat grill or broiler.

2. In a medium bowl, combine lemon juice, zest, sesame oil, chili sauce, and cayenne pepper; mix well. Add scallops and toss to coat. Let stand for 15 minutes.

3. Thread a skewer through one end of the bacon, then add a scallop. Curve the bacon around the scallop and thread onto the skewer, so it surrounds the scallop halfway. Repeat with 3–4 more scallops and the bacon slice. Repeat with remaining scallops and bacon.

4. Grill or broil 6" from heat source for 3–5 minutes per side, until bacon is crisp and scallops are cooked and opaque. Serve immediately.

♥ **PER SERVING** Calories: 173.65 | Fat: 6.48 g | Saturated fat: 1.51 g | Sodium: 266.64 mg | Cholesterol: 46.20 mg

Shrimp Toasts

These tasty bites are a gourmet addition to any summer party. Try experimenting with different herbs and spices to create your own signature appetizer.

INGREDIENTS | SERVES 48

1 pound shrimp, peeled and deveined

¼ cup minced green onions

2 tablespoons minced fresh cilantro

1 teaspoon minced garlic

1 teaspoon minced jalapeño pepper

1 large egg white

1 tablespoon nonfat dry milk

4 ounces cream cheese, cut into pieces

½ cup plain nonfat yogurt

12 (1-ounce) slices Basic White Bread (see Chapter 16), crusts removed

Spectrum Naturals Extra Virgin Olive Spray Oil with Garlic Flavor

Spectrum Naturals Canola Spray Oil with Butter Flavor

Saving Some Steps

There's no reason to take the time to remove the crusts from homemade bread slice by slice. Before you slice the bread, cut off the crusts. Then slice the bread into 1-ounce pieces.

1. Preheat the oven to 375°F.

2. In a food processor, combine the shrimp, green onions, cilantro, garlic, jalapeño, egg white, and nonfat dry milk; process until smooth. Add cubes of cream cheese; pulse to incorporate. Add yogurt; pulse just until incorporated, being careful not to overprocess.

3. To shorten baking time and help ensure bread is crisp in center, first toast it; then spray bottom of each slice with a light amount of garlic-flavored spray oil.

4. Evenly divide shrimp mixture between slices of bread, spreading it on nonsprayed side of bread and making sure to spread it to edges.

5. Place bread slices shrimp mixture-side up on a baking sheet treated with nonstick spray or covered with nonstick foil. Lightly spray tops of bread with butter-flavored spray oil.

6. Bake 10–15 minutes, or until bread is crisp and shrimp topping bubbles and is lightly browned. Use a pizza cutter or serrated knife to cut each slice of bread into 4 equal pieces. Arrange on a tray or platter, and serve immediately.

♥ **PER SERVING** Calories: 42.35 | Fat: 1.33 g | Saturated fat: 0.60 g | Sodium: 49.03 mg | Cholesterol: 17.02 mg

Simple Tomato Sauce

This sauce can be used as a base in a number of recipes. Try it on pizza, with spaghetti and meatballs, or to dip a panini sandwich in.

INGREDIENTS | SERVES 12

½ cup extra-virgin olive oil

1 large sweet onion, chopped

2 cloves garlic, minced

1 large stalk celery, finely chopped

1 large carrot, peeled and grated

¼ teaspoon freshly ground black pepper

⅛ teaspoon mustard powder

1 (14.5-ounce) can Muir Glen Organic No-Salt-Added Diced Tomatoes

¼ teaspoon granulated sugar, or to taste

⅛ teaspoon dried lemon granules, crushed

1 (15-ounce) can Muir Glen Organic No-Salt-Added Tomato Sauce

1 (28-ounce) can Muir Glen Organic No-Salt-Added Tomato Purée

2 dried bay leaves

½ teaspoon dried oregano, crushed

½ teaspoon dried basil, crushed

Pinch red pepper flakes

1 teaspoon garlic powder (optional)

1 teaspoon onion powder (optional)

4 tablespoons unsalted butter or fine extra-virgin olive oil (optional)

Leveraging Lycopene

There's evidence that the nutritional benefits of tomatoes increase when you cook them, because cooking makes lycopene more available to the body than when tomatoes are eaten raw. Lycopene is the antioxidant that gives tomatoes their red color; recent studies indicate lycopene helps lessen the chance of certain cancers.

1. In a large, deep nonstick sauté pan, heat the oil over medium-high heat. Add the onion and garlic; sauté until soft and translucent, about 5–10 minutes. Add the celery, carrots, black pepper, and mustard powder; mix well. Sauté for 5 minutes.

2. Drain juice from diced tomatoes; reserve. Add drained tomatoes to the pot; sauté until all vegetables are soft, about 5–10 minutes.

3. In a food processor, add sautéed tomato mixture and process until smooth. Return to the pan.

4. Add reserved juice from tomatoes, sugar, lemon granules, tomato sauce, tomato purée, bay leaves, oregano, basil, and red pepper flakes; reduce heat and simmer, uncovered, for 45 minutes.

5. Remove the bay leaves and check for seasoning; add garlic and onion powders at this time, if desired. Simmer for an additional 15 minutes, or until thick. If the sauce tastes too acidic, add a little bit more sugar or some fresh or dried thyme, a pinch at a time; if you're not watching your fat and cholesterol, you can also mellow the flavor by whisking in some unsalted butter, 1 tablespoon at a time; otherwise, use fine extra-virgin olive oil.

6. If you are not using all the sauce immediately, allow it to cool completely and pour 1 cup portions into freezer containers; it will keep in the freezer for up to 6 months.

♥ **PER SERVING** Calories: 88.33 | Fat: 4.54 g | Saturated fat: 0.62 g | Sodium: 57.72 mg | Cholesterol: 0.00 mg

Low-Fat Tomato Sauce

This recipe may be low in fat, but it's full of flavor.

INGREDIENTS | SERVES 12

Spectrum Naturals Extra-Virgin Olive Spray Oil

1 large sweet onion, chopped

2 cloves garlic, minced

1 large stalk celery, finely chopped

1 large carrot, peeled and grated

1 dried bay leaf

1 (14.5-ounce) can Muir Glen Organic No-Salt-Added Diced Tomatoes

½ teaspoon dried oregano, crushed

½ teaspoon dried basil, crushed

Pinch red pepper flakes

⅛ teaspoon mustard powder

1 teaspoon granulated sugar, or to taste

⅛ teaspoon dried lemon granules, crushed

1 (15-ounce) can Muir Glen Organic No-Salt-Added Tomato Sauce

1 (28-ounce) can Muir Glen Organic No-Salt-Added Tomato Purée

1 teaspoon garlic powder

1 teaspoon onion powder

2 teaspoons extra-virgin olive oil

It Only Takes a Tad

A pinch of sugar is a wonderful flavor enhancer and helps cut the acidity in cooked tomato sauces and soups.

1. In a large, covered microwave-safe casserole dish treated with olive spray oil, add the onion, garlic, celery, carrots, and bay leaf.

2. Drain juice from diced tomatoes; reserve. Add tomatoes to dish; mix well. Cover and microwave on high 5 minutes, turning dish halfway through cooking time.

3. Carefully remove cover; stir in oregano, basil, red pepper flakes, mustard powder, sugar, and lemon granules. Cover and let rest 3 minutes.

4. Carefully remove cover and check that onion is transparent; if not, microwave on high in additional 1-minute increments until all vegetables are cooked and soft. Remove bay leaf.

5. In food processor, add sautéed tomato mixture; process until smooth.

6. Bring a large, deep nonstick sauté pan treated with spray oil to temperature over low heat. Add puréed tomato-vegetable mixture, reserved tomato juice, tomato sauce, and tomato purée; reduce heat and simmer, uncovered, for 45 minutes.

7. Add garlic and onion powders; simmer additional 15 minutes, or until thick. Whisk in extra-virgin olive oil. If the sauce tastes too acidic, add a little bit more sugar or thyme, a pinch at a time.

8. If you are not using all the sauce immediately, allow it to cool completely and pour 1 cup portions into freezer containers; it will keep for up to 6 months.

♥ **PER SERVING** Calories: 56.19 | Fat: 0.79 g | Saturated fat: 0.11 g | Sodium: 57.73 mg | Cholesterol: 0.00 mg

Spinach Ravioli in Tomato Mushroom Sauce

This recipe is a lighter version of classic ravioli. It's so delicious, your family won't know it's low in calories!

Skipping the Salt—Cooked Pasta Instructions

Instead of adding salt to the water when you boil pasta, as called for on most packages, skip the salt and instead add 1 tablespoon fresh lemon juice or ¼ teaspoon crushed dried lemon granules and ¼ teaspoon mustard powder to the water. It provides great flavor without the sodium.

1. In a small bowl, add spinach, ricotta, nutmeg, and 4 teaspoons of Parmesan; mix well.

2. To fill egg roll wrappers, line half of wrappers on a cutting board. Brush with egg and water mixture. Using a teaspoon, arrange a dollop of filling on each wrapper. Place another wrapper directly on top, pressing around filling and sealing edges. Crimp edges with a fork. Place onto a floured baking sheet; keep covered with a damp cotton towel.

3. Bring a large, deep nonstick sauté pan to temperature over medium heat. Add 3 teaspoons of olive oil. Add mushrooms; sauté for 3–5 minutes.

4. Stir in tomato sauce and any remaining egg-water mixture; reduce heat and keep warm.

5. In a large pot, bring 4 quarts of water to a boil; add lemon juice and remaining 1 teaspoon oil. Carefully add small batches of ravioli, about 3–4 at a time. This will prevent them from crowding in pot and sticking together.

6. Cook 2–3 minutes. Using a spider strainer or slotted spoon, carefully remove ravioli; place on a plate. Tent with foil to keep warm while cooking remaining ravioli.

7. Divide cooked ravioli between 4 serving plates. Top with sauce; sprinkle with 1 teaspoon of remaining Parmesan. Serve immediately.

♥ **PER SERVING** Calories: 387.39 | Fat: 11.31 g | Saturated Fat: 3.11 g | Sodium: 598.49 mg | Cholesterol: 119.45 mg

Spinach Pasta in Tuna Alfredo Sauce

Usually, any recipe with "alfredo" in the title translates to a high-fat, high-calorie dish. This version lightens up the sauce for guilt-free dining.

INGREDIENTS | SERVES 4

1 cup nonfat cottage cheese

1 tablespoon skim milk

⅛ teaspoon freshly ground black pepper

⅛ teaspoon mustard powder

2 teaspoons olive oil

1 clove minced garlic

2 (6-ounce) cans Chicken of the Sea Very Low Sodium Tuna, drained

⅛ cup dry white wine

¼ cup freshly grated Parmesan cheese

4 cups cooked spinach pasta

1. In a food processor or blender, add the cottage cheese, skim milk, pepper, and mustard powder; process until smooth. Set aside.

2. Bring the olive oil to temperature in a large, deep nonstick sauté pan over medium heat. Add the garlic; sauté for 1 minute.

3. Stir in the tuna; sauté for 1 more minute. Add wine to the skillet; bring to a boil.

4. Lower the heat and add creamed cottage cheese; bring to temperature, being careful not to boil the cream.

5. Stir in Parmesan; continue to heat sauce another minute, stirring constantly. Add pasta; toss with the sauce.

6. Divide into 4 equal servings; serve immediately, topped with additional freshly ground pepper, if desired.

♥ **PER SERVING** Calories: 297.96 | Fat: 4.04 g | Saturated fat: 1.52 g | Sodium: 167.31 mg | Cholesterol: 26.23 mg

Easy Chicken Lo Mein

This is a healthier version of the takeout classic—you'll consume less fat and calories and a fraction of the sodium of typical restaurant lo mein dishes.

INGREDIENTS | SERVES 4

⅛ teaspoon Minor's Low Sodium Chicken Base

½ cup water

2 (10-ounce) packages Cascadian Farm Organic Frozen Chinese Stir-Fry Vegetables

1 tablespoon freeze-dried shallots

1 pound cooked dark- and light-meat chicken

⅛ cup Mr. Spice Ginger Stir-Fry Sauce, or to taste

1 pound no-salt-added oat bran pasta

1 teaspoon lemon juice

⅛ teaspoon mustard powder

1 teaspoon cornstarch

¼ teaspoon toasted sesame oil

4 thinly sliced scallions (optional)

Bragg Liquid Aminos or other low-sodium soy sauce (optional)

Great Grains

If you prefer to serve the stir-fry over brown rice—or another grain, like quinoa—simply add some lemon juice and mustard powder to the cooking water instead of the salt suggested on the package.

1. In a large microwave-safe bowl, add chicken base and water; microwave on high 30 seconds. Stir to dissolve base into water. Add vegetables and shallots; microwave on high 3–5 minutes, depending on how you prefer your vegetables cooked. Drain some of the broth into a small nonstick sauté pan and set aside.

2. Add chicken and stir-fry sauce to vegetables; stir well. Cover and set aside.

3. In a large pot, bring amount of water noted on pasta package to a boil, omitting salt. Add pasta, lemon juice, and mustard powder.

4. In a small cup or bowl, add 1 tablespoon of water to cornstarch; whisk to make a slurry.

5. Bring reserved broth in sauté pan to a boil over medium-high heat. Whisk in slurry; cook at least 1 minute (to remove the raw cornstarch taste), stirring constantly. Once mixture thickens, remove from heat; add toasted sesame oil to broth mixture, then whisk again.

6. Pour thickened broth mixture over vegetables and chicken; toss to mix. Cover and microwave at 70 percent power 2 minutes, or until chicken is heated through.

7. Drain pasta; add it to chicken-vegetable mixture, and stir to combine. Divide among 4 plates. Garnish with chopped scallion, and serve with Bragg Liquid Aminos at the table, if desired.

♥ **PER SERVING** Calories: 406.19 | Fat: 5.38 g | Saturated fat: 1.35 g | Sodium: 138.59 mg | Cholesterol: 96.44 mg

Chickpeas in Lettuce Wraps

*This delicious creamy and flavorful spread is also great
on toasted bread or used as an appetizer dip.*

INGREDIENTS | SERVES 6–8

1 (15-ounce) can no-salt chickpeas

3 tablespoons olive oil

3 tablespoons lemon juice

3 cloves garlic, minced

1 tablespoon chopped fresh mint

½ cup diced red onion

8 lettuce leaves

1 cup chopped tomatoes

1 cup chopped yellow bell pepper

1. Drain the chickpeas; rinse, and drain again. Place half in a blender or food processor. Add olive oil, lemon juice, garlic, and mint; blend or process until smooth.

2. Place in a medium bowl; stir in remaining chickpeas and red onion until combined.

3. To make wraps, place lettuce leaves on work surface. Divide chickpea mixture among leaves and top with tomatoes and bell pepper. Roll up, folding in sides, to enclose filling. Serve immediately.

♥ **PER SERVING** Calories: 148.96 | Fat: 6.56 g | Saturated fat: 0.87 g | Sodium: 6.80 mg | Cholesterol: 0.00 mg

Zesty Herbed Dilly Beans

This is a great side to serve at your next barbecue; it's cool, crisp, and refreshing.

INGREDIENTS | SERVES 16

1 (16-ounce) package Cascadian Farms Organic Frozen Green Beans, thawed

¾ cup apple cider vinegar

¾ cup water

¼ teaspoon cayenne pepper or dried red pepper flakes

2 cloves garlic, minced

2 teaspoons dill seeds

1 teaspoon dried dill weed

½ teaspoon salt

1. Put the green beans in a glass jar or other covered container large enough to hold the beans and vinegar mixture.

2. In a medium nonreactive saucepan over high heat, bring the vinegar and water to a boil. Stir in the cayenne pepper, garlic, dill seeds and weed, and salt. Pour the vinegar mixture over the green beans. Allow to cool to room temperature.

3. Cover and refrigerate for 24 hours before serving. Store leftovers in the refrigerator. Use within 1 week.

♥ **PER SERVING** Calories: 13.19 | Fat: 0.05 g | Saturated fat: 0.00 g | Sodium: 73.04 mg | Cholesterol: 0.00 mg

Red-Bean Salad with Taco Chips

*Low-fat taco chips are usually baked. Read labels carefully and pick
a version that is low-fat and made with whole grain.*

INGREDIENTS | SERVES 6

¼ cup lime juice

½ cup low-fat sour cream

½ cup plain yogurt

½ teaspoon crushed red pepper flakes

1 red onion, chopped

2 jalapeño peppers, minced

1 green bell pepper, chopped

3 stalks celery, chopped

4 cups Beans for Soup (see Chapter 13)

6 cups shredded lettuce

½ cup pumpkin seeds

2 cups crushed low-fat taco chips

1. In a large bowl, combine lime juice, sour cream, yogurt, pepper flakes, onion, and jalapeño peppers; mix well. Add bell pepper, celery, and beans; mix well. This can be chilled, well covered, until ready to eat.

2. When ready to serve, arrange lettuce on a serving platter; spoon bean mixture over top. Sprinkle with pumpkin seeds and crushed taco chips, and serve immediately.

♥ **PER SERVING** Calories: 324.28 | Fat: 8.60 g | Saturated fat: 2.83 g | Dietary fiber: 13.31 g | Sodium: 204.12 mg | Cholesterol: 10.03 mg

Beans

Any type of bean or legume can be substituted for another. You could use kidney beans, black beans, Great Northern beans, navy beans, black-eyed peas, pink beans, or chickpeas in this delicious salad. Beans are very high in fiber, help lower cholesterol, and have been a major protein source for populations around the world for centuries.

Black-Eyed Pea Salad

*Black-eyed peas contain pectin, another soluble fiber that helps
reduce cholesterol levels. And they're delicious!*

INGREDIENTS | SERVES 6–8

1 (16-ounce) package dried black-eyed peas
8 cups cold water
1 cup plain yogurt
¼ cup olive oil
¼ cup Dijon mustard
1 teaspoon dried thyme leaves
¼ teaspoon salt
⅛ teaspoon pepper
2 green bell peppers, chopped
1 red bell pepper, chopped
1 red onion, finely chopped
½ cup crumbled goat cheese

1. Pick over peas and rinse; drain well. Place in a large pot; cover with cold water, cover with pot lid, and let stand overnight.

2. In the morning, drain and rinse peas; cover with cold water again. Bring to a boil, then reduce heat; simmer 75–85 minutes, until tender.

3. In large bowl, combine yogurt, olive oil, mustard, thyme, salt, and pepper; mix well. When peas are cooked, drain well and add to yogurt mixture along with peppers and red onion.

4. Toss gently to coat; sprinkle with goat cheese. Cover and refrigerate 4–6 hours before serving.

♥ **PER SERVING** Calories: 174.84 | Fat: 9.30 g | Saturated fat: 2.37 g | Dietary fiber: 4.37 g | Sodium: 212.18 mg | Cholesterol: 5.10 mg

Tuna-Pasta Salad

Celery and carrots add a great crunch to this sweet pasta salad.

INGREDIENTS | **SERVES 2**

1 (6-ounce) can Chicken of the Sea 50% less sodium tuna, drained

1 tablespoon Hellmann's or Best Foods Real Mayonnaise

1 tablespoon nonfat yogurt

2 teaspoons sweet pickle relish

1 teaspoon cane sugar

1 teaspoon champagne or white wine vinegar

2 cups cooked spaghetti, cooked in unsalted water

½ cup diced celery

10 medium-size baby carrots, sliced

½ teaspoon Spice House Salt-Free Sunny Paris Seasoning (optional)

Chopped fresh or freeze-dried chives, scallions, or freeze-dried green onions for garnish (optional)

1. Combine the tuna, mayonnaise, yogurt, relish, sugar, and vinegar in a bowl; stir until well mixed.

2. Add spaghetti, celery, and carrots; toss to mix.

3. Mix in optional seasoning, if using. Refrigerate until needed. Garnish with chopped chives, if desired.

♥ **PER SERVING** Calories: 376.31 | Fat: 3.72 g | Saturated fat: 0.47 g | Sodium: 305.56 mg | Cholesterol: 39.56 mg

CHAPTER 16

Heart-Healthy Bread, Dessert, and Dressing Recipes

Basic White Bread

This bread can be used in a number of recipes. Try it for sandwiches, with salads, in appetizers—get creative!

INGREDIENTS | SERVES 24

1 teaspoon active dry yeast

1 teaspoon granulated sugar

1⅓ cups lukewarm water (about 105°F)

2 tablespoons extra-virgin olive oil

1 teaspoon fine sea salt

4 cups unbleached bread flour

1. **To make the dough:** In the bowl of a heavy-duty electric mixer fitted with a dough-hook attachment, combine yeast, sugar, and water. Mix on lowest speed to blend. Let stand until the yeast bubbles, about 5 minutes.

2. Add the oil and salt; mix on lowest speed to blend. Add 3 cups of flour; resume mixing adding remaining flour a little at a time until flour has been absorbed and dough forms a ball and pulls away from side of mixer.

3. Increase mixer to the speed recommended by the manufacturer for kneading dough; mix until dough is soft and has a satiny sheen, about 4–5 minutes.

4. Transfer dough to a bowl that has a capacity 3 times the size of ball of dough; cover tightly with plastic wrap and place in refrigerator. Let dough rise until doubled or tripled in bulk, 8–12 hours. Dough can be refrigerated 2–3 days.

5. **To bake bread:** Treat a bread pan with olive oil or nonstick cooking spray. Remove dough from refrigerator; punch down. If necessary, rub a little olive oil on your hands and work dough by folding it over itself a few times, pinching resulting "seam" together.

6. Arrange in pan seam-side down. Brush a little oil over top of dough. Cover with a cotton towel; set in a warm place and let rise until doubled in size.

7. Preheat oven to 350°F. Cut 1–2 slits in top of dough. Bake 30–40 minutes, or until bread has a hollow sound when thumped. Cool in pan, remove, and cool on wire rack.

♥ **PER SERVING** Calories: 86.95 | Fat: 1.34 g | Saturated fat: 0.19 g | Sodium: 97.40 mg | Cholesterol: 0.00 mg

Navajo Chili Bread

Serve this spicy quick bread warm with a pot of Three-Bean Chili
(see Chapter 13) for a warming dinner on a cold day.

INGREDIENTS | **YIELDS 1 LOAF; 12 SERVINGS**

3 tablespoons olive oil

½ cup minced onion

2 cloves garlic, minced

2 jalapeño peppers, minced

½ cup finely chopped red bell pepper

1¼ cups all-purpose flour

1 cup yellow cornmeal

⅛ teaspoon salt

1 teaspoon baking powder

½ teaspoon baking soda

2 teaspoons chili powder

½ cup liquid egg substitute

¾ cup buttermilk

2 tablespoons molasses

½ cup shredded pepper jack cheese

1. Preheat oven to 375°F. Spray a 9" square glass baking dish with nonstick cooking spray containing flour, and set aside.

2. In a small saucepan, heat olive oil over medium heat. Add onion, garlic, jalapeño, and red bell pepper; cook and stir until crisp-tender, about 4 minutes. Remove from heat.

3. In a large bowl, combine flour, cornmeal, salt, baking powder, baking soda, and chili powder; mix to combine.

4. Add egg substitute, buttermilk, and molasses to vegetables in saucepan; beat to combine. Stir into flour mixture until combined; fold in cheese.

5. Pour batter into prepared pan. Bake 30–40 minutes, or until bread is light golden-brown and toothpick inserted in center comes out clean. Let cool for 15 minutes, then serve.

♥ **PER SERVING** Calories: 223.97 | Fat: 7.59 g | Saturated fat: 2.11 g | Sodium: 232.04 mg | Cholesterol: 6.54 mg

Banana-Blueberry Oatmeal Bread

*Quick breads are easy to make. Their flavor and texture usually gets better
if allowed to stand, covered, overnight at room temperature.*

INGREDIENTS | YIELDS 1 LOAF; 12 SERVINGS

1 (3-ounce) package light cream cheese, softened

¼ cup brown sugar

¼ cup sugar

2 bananas, mashed

1 egg

2 egg whites

¼ cup orange juice

1 cup all-purpose flour

½ cup whole-wheat flour

1 teaspoon baking powder

1 teaspoon baking soda

1 cup blueberries

½ cup regular oatmeal

1. Preheat the oven to 350°F. Spray a 9" × 5" loaf pan with nonstick cooking spray containing flour; set aside.

2. In a large bowl, combine cream cheese, brown sugar, and sugar; beat until fluffy. Beat in mashed bananas, then add egg, egg whites, and orange juice; beat until smooth.

3. Stir together flour, whole-wheat flour, baking powder, and baking soda; add to batter, and stir just until combined. Fold in blueberries and oatmeal; pour into prepared loaf pan.

4. Bake 50–60 minutes, or until bread is deep golden-brown and toothpick inserted in center comes out clean. Remove from pan, and cool on wire rack.

♥ **PER SERVING** Calories: 165.78 | Fat: 2.43 g | Saturated fat: 1.05 g | Sodium: 173.82 mg | Cholesterol: 21.59 mg

Fresh or Frozen Fruit?

When baking, you can usually use either fresh or frozen fruit. If using frozen, do not thaw before adding it to the batter, or it will add too much liquid and color or stain the bread. Use frozen fruits that are dry-packed, with no added sugar or other ingredients.

Zucchini-Walnut Bread

When your garden is overflowing with zucchini in late summer, make several batches of this bread and freeze for the long winter months.

INGREDIENTS | **YIELDS 1 LOAF; 12 SERVINGS**

¼ cup canola oil

¼ cup sugar

½ cup brown sugar

1 egg

2 egg whites

½ cup orange juice

2 teaspoons vanilla

1 cup grated zucchini

1 teaspoon grated lemon zest

2 tablespoons wheat germ

1 cup all-purpose flour

1 cup whole-wheat flour

1 teaspoon baking powder

½ teaspoon baking soda

⅛ teaspoon salt

1 teaspoon cinnamon

¼ teaspoon cloves

½ cup chopped walnuts

1. Preheat the oven to 350°F. Spray a 9" × 5" loaf pan with nonstick cooking spray containing flour; set aside.

2. In a large bowl, combine oil, sugar, brown sugar, egg, egg whites, orange juice, and vanilla; beat until smooth. Stir in zucchini, lemon zest, and wheat germ.

3. Sift together flour, whole-wheat flour, baking powder, baking soda, salt, cinnamon, and cloves; add to oil mixture. Stir just until combined; fold in walnuts. Pour into prepared pan.

4. Bake 55–65 minutes, or until bread is golden-brown and toothpick inserted in center comes out clean. Remove from pan, and let cool on wire rack.

♥ **PER SERVING** Calories: 217.46 | Fat: 8.48 g | Saturated fat: 0.70 g | Sodium: 127.63 mg | Cholesterol: 17.63 mg

Carrot-Oatmeal Bread

This bread is like carrot cake, but not as sweet. Try it in a chicken salad sandwich!

INGREDIENTS | **YIELDS 1 LOAF; 12 SERVINGS**

1½ cups finely chopped carrots
1 cup water
1½ cups all-purpose flour
¾ cup oatmeal
2 tablespoons oat bran
½ cup brown sugar
⅓ cup sugar
½ teaspoon salt
1 teaspoon baking powder
½ teaspoon baking soda
½ teaspoon cinnamon
½ teaspoon ginger
⅔ cup applesauce
¼ cup canola oil
2 egg whites
½ cup chopped walnuts

1. Preheat the oven to 350°F. Spray a 9" × 5" loaf pan with nonstick cooking spray containing flour; set aside.

2. In a small saucepan, combine carrots and water; bring to a boil. Reduce heat and simmer 5–7 minutes, or until carrots are tender. Drain carrots; mash until smooth. Set aside.

3. In a large bowl, combine flour, oatmeal, oat bran, brown sugar, sugar, salt, baking powder, baking soda, cinnamon, and ginger; mix well.

4. In a medium bowl, combine mashed carrots, applesauce, canola oil, and egg whites; beat well. Stir into dry ingredients until blended; fold in walnuts.

5. Pour batter into prepared pan. Bake 55–65 minutes, or until bread is deep golden-brown and toothpick inserted in center comes out clean. Remove from pan, and let cool on wire rack.

♥ **PER SERVING** Calories: 241.05 | Fat: 8.56 g | Saturated fat: 0.66 g | Sodium: 107.36 mg | Cholesterol: 0.00 mg

Apple-Cranberry Nut Bread

This fragrant bread is a wonderful use for fall apples. Serve it for a quick breakfast.

INGREDIENTS | **YIELDS 1 LOAF; 12 SERVINGS**

2 apples, peeled and chopped

¼ cup sugar

½ cup brown sugar

¼ cup canola oil

1 egg

2 teaspoons vanilla

1 cup apple juice, divided

1¼ cups all-purpose flour

¾ cup whole-wheat flour

1 teaspoon baking powder

½ teaspoon baking soda

1 teaspoon cinnamon

½ cup dried cranberries

½ cup fresh chopped cranberries

½ cup chopped walnuts

1 cup powdered sugar

1. Preheat the oven to 350°F. Spray a 9" × 5" loaf pan with nonstick cooking spray containing flour; set aside.

2. In a large bowl, combine apples and ¼ cup sugar; let stand 15 minutes. Add brown sugar, oil, egg, vanilla, and ⅔ cup apple juice; mix well.

3. In a medium bowl, combine flour, whole-wheat flour, baking powder and soda, cinnamon, both types of cranberries, and walnuts; stir to mix. Add to apple mixture; stir until blended.

4. Pour into prepared pan. Bake 55–65 minutes, or until bread is golden-brown and toothpick inserted in center comes out clean. Remove from pan, and place on wire rack.

5. In small bowl, combine remaining 1/3 cup apple juice and powdered sugar; mix well. Drizzle over warm bread; let stand until cool.

♥ **PER SERVING** Calories: 268.90 | Fat: 8.39 g | Saturated fat: 0.68 g | Sodium: 93.75 mg | Cholesterol: 17.63 mg

Savory Herb Muffins

These little muffins are delicious served with soup for lunch on a cold day.

INGREDIENTS | YIELDS 12 MUFFINS

1 cup buttermilk

1 egg

2 egg whites

5 tablespoons canola oil

2 tablespoons chopped fresh rosemary leaves

2 teaspoons fresh thyme leaves

2 tablespoons chopped flat-leaf parsley

¼ teaspoon dried marjoram

¼ cup grated Parmesan cheese

½ cup cornmeal

1¼ cups all-purpose flour

½ cup whole-wheat flour

1 teaspoon baking powder

1 teaspoon baking soda

1. Preheat the oven to 375°F. Place paper liners into 12 muffin cups; set aside.

2. In a large bowl, combine buttermilk, egg, egg whites, canola oil, all the herbs, Parmesan, and cornmeal; mix well until combined. Add flour, whole-wheat flour, baking powder, and baking soda; stir just until dry ingredients are moistened.

3. Fill prepared muffin cups ⅔ full. Bake 20–25 minutes, or until muffins are light golden-brown and set. Remove from muffin cups, and serve warm.

♥ **PER SERVING** Calories: 161.90 | Fat: 7.19 g | Saturated fat: 1.05 g | Sodium: 204.07 mg | Cholesterol: 20.27 mg

Rosemary

Rosemary is one of the herbs believed to reduce arterial inflammation. Try to find fresh rosemary; dried rosemary is so stiff and brittle it has to be chopped very fine or it can be difficult to swallow. To use fresh rosemary, pull the thin leaves backward from the stem, then pile up and chop with a chef's knife.

Good Morning Muffins

These moist muffins are packed with fiber and nutrition. Serve them warm with some whipped honey. Yum.

INGREDIENTS | **YIELDS 18 MUFFINS**

1 cup all-purpose flour

1 cup whole-wheat flour

2 tablespoons oat bran

2 tablespoons ground flaxseed

½ cup sugar

½ cup brown sugar

2 teaspoons cinnamon

¼ teaspoon nutmeg

1½ teaspoons baking powder

1 teaspoon baking soda

2 apples, peeled and chopped

1 cup grated carrots

½ cup applesauce

1 egg

1 egg white

¼ cup low-fat sour cream

¼ cup canola oil

2 teaspoons vanilla

1 cup dried cranberries

1 cup chopped walnuts

1. Preheat the oven to 375°F. Line 18 muffin cups with paper liners; set aside.

2. In a large bowl, combine flour, whole-wheat flour, oat bran, flaxseed, sugar, brown sugar, cinnamon, nutmeg, baking powder, and baking soda; mix well.

3. In a medium bowl, combine apples, carrots, applesauce, egg, egg white, sour cream, canola oil, and vanilla; beat to combine. Add to flour mixture; stir just until dry ingredients are moistened. Fold in cranberries and walnuts.

4. Fill prepared muffin cups ¾ full. Bake 15–25 minutes, or until muffins are golden-brown and toothpick inserted in center comes out clean. Remove from muffin cups and cool on wire rack.

♥ **PER SERVING** Calories: 210.22 | Fat: 8.48 g | Saturated fat: 0.86 g | Sodium: 116.29 mg | Cholesterol: 13.06 mg

Cranberry-Orange Bread

Cranberry and orange is an irresistible combination. Serve this bread with low-fat fruit-flavored cream cheese spread.

INGREDIENTS | YIELDS 1 LOAF: 12 SERVINGS

¾ cup orange juice

2 tablespoons frozen orange juice concentrate, thawed

½ teaspoon almond extract

¼ cup canola oil

1 egg

⅓ cup sugar

½ cup brown sugar

1 teaspoon grated orange zest

1½ cups all-purpose flour

¾ cup whole-wheat flour

1 teaspoon baking soda

1 teaspoon baking powder

2 cups chopped cranberries

½ cup chopped hazelnuts

1. Preheat the oven to 350°F. Spray a 9" × 5" loaf pan with nonstick cooking spray containing flour; set aside.

2. In a medium bowl, combine orange juice, orange juice concentrate, almond extract, canola oil, egg, sugar, brown sugar, and orange zest; beat to combine.

3. In a large bowl, combine flour, whole-wheat flour, baking soda, and baking powder; mix. Make a well in the center of the flour mixture; pour in orange juice mixture. Stir just until dry ingredients are moistened. Fold in cranberries and hazelnuts.

4. Pour into prepared pan. Bake 55–65 minutes, or until bread is golden-brown and toothpick inserted in center comes out clean. Remove from pan, and let cool on wire rack.

♥ **PER SERVING** Calories: 232.48 | Fat: 8.24 g | Saturated fat: 0.72 g | Sodium: 145.81 mg | Cholesterol: 17.63 mg

Self-Rising Flour

If you're watching your sodium intake, do not use self-rising flour. On average, it contains 1½ teaspoons of baking powder and ½ teaspoon of salt per cup, which together add more than 1,700 mg of sodium. Just use whole-wheat or all-purpose flour, adding 1 teaspoon baking powder and a pinch of salt per cup.

Cheddar-Herb Biscuits

*These biscuits have to be served hot from the oven! Offer a nonfat
cream cheese spread flavored with more herbs.*

INGREDIENTS | YIELDS 8 BISCUITS

1½ cups all-purpose flour

½ cup whole-wheat flour

1½ teaspoons baking powder

½ teaspoon baking soda

¼ teaspoon garlic salt

¼ cup canola oil

1 egg white

⅔ cup buttermilk

1 cup grated low-fat extra-sharp
Cheddar cheese

1 tablespoon chopped fresh rosemary

1 tablespoon fresh thyme leaves

1 tablespoon butter or plant sterol
margarine, melted

1 tablespoon chopped flat-leaf parsley

1. Preheat the oven to 400°F. Line a cookie sheet with parchment paper and set aside.

2. In a large bowl, combine flour, whole-wheat flour, baking powder, baking soda, and garlic salt; mix well.

3. In a small bowl, combine oil, egg white, and buttermilk. Add all at once to dry ingredients; stir just until moistened.

4. Fold in cheese, rosemary, and thyme leaves. Drop into 8 mounds onto prepared cookie sheet; bake for 15–20 minutes, or until biscuits are light golden-brown.

5. In a small microwave-safe bowl, melt butter. Add parsley; stir well. Brush over hot biscuits. Remove biscuits to wire rack to cool slightly before serving.

♥ **PER SERVING** Calories: 218.86 | Fat: 9.80 g | Saturated fat: 2.18 g | Sodium: 272.53 mg | Cholesterol: 7.60 mg

Whole-Grain Cornbread

*Cornbread should be eaten hot from the oven. Instead of slathering it with butter,
spread with whipped honey or top with Super Spicy Salsa (see Chapter 13).*

INGREDIENTS | SERVES 9

¾ cup all-purpose flour
½ cup whole-wheat flour
¼ cup brown sugar
2 teaspoons baking powder
1 teaspoon baking soda
1 cup cornmeal
⅓ cup oat bran
1 egg
2 egg whites
¼ cup honey
1 cup buttermilk
¼ cup canola oil

1. Preheat the oven to 400°F. Spray a 9" square pan with nonstick cooking spray containing flour; set aside.

2. In a large mixing bowl, combine flour, whole-wheat flour, brown sugar, baking powder, baking soda, cornmeal, and oat bran; mix well.

3. In a small bowl, combine egg, egg whites, honey, buttermilk, and canola oil; beat to combine. Add to dry ingredients; stir just until mixed.

4. Spoon into prepared pan; smooth top. Bake for 25–35 minutes, or until bread is golden brown.

♥ **PER SERVING** Calories: 252.79 | Fat: 7.58 g | Saturated fat: 0.87 g | Sodium: 272.96 mg | Cholesterol: 24.59 mg

Oat-Bran Date Muffins

*Dates contain lots of soluble fiber and are naturally sweet.
Keep some Medjool dates on hand for snacking.*

INGREDIENTS | YIELDS 12 MUFFINS

1¼ cups all-purpose flour
½ cup rolled oats
¼ cup oat bran
1½ teaspoons baking powder
1 teaspoon baking soda
⅓ cup brown sugar
1 egg
¼ cup canola oil
⅓ cup applesauce
1 teaspoon grated orange zest
1 cup finely chopped dates
½ cup chopped hazelnuts

1. Preheat the oven to 350°F. Line 12 muffin cups with paper liners; set aside. In large bowl, combine flour, oats, oat bran, baking powder, baking soda, and brown sugar.

2. In a medium bowl, combine egg, canola oil, applesauce, and orange zest; beat to combine. Add to dry ingredients; stir just until moistened. Fold in dates and hazelnuts.

3. Fill prepared muffin cups ⅔ full. Bake for 25–35 minutes, or until muffins are set and toothpick inserted in center comes out clean. Remove from muffin cups to wire racks to cool.

♥ **PER SERVING** Calories: 232.40 | Fat: 8.66 g | Saturated fat: 0.80 g | Sodium: 159.46 mg | Cholesterol: 17.63 mg

Cranberry-Cornmeal Muffins

Masa harina is corn flour; it's not the same as cornmeal. You can find it in the international foods aisle of the supermarket.

INGREDIENTS | YIELDS 12 MUFFINS

½ cup cornmeal

½ cup masa harina

1 cup all-purpose flour

2 tablespoons crushed flaxseed

¼ cup brown sugar

1 teaspoon baking powder

1 teaspoon baking soda

1 egg

¼ cup canola oil

1 cup buttermilk

1 teaspoon grated orange zest

2 tablespoons honey

1 teaspoon vanilla

⅓ cup chopped cranberries

⅓ cup dried cranberries

1. Preheat the oven to 400°F. Line 12 muffin cups with paper liners; set aside.

2. In a large bowl, combine cornmeal, masa harina, flour, flaxseed, brown sugar, baking powder, and baking soda; mix well.

3. In a small bowl, combine egg, oil, buttermilk, orange zest, honey, and vanilla; beat to combine. Add to dry ingredients; stir just until moistened. Add chopped and dried cranberries.

4. Fill muffin cups ⅔ full. Bake for 15–22 minutes, or until toothpick inserted in center comes out clean. Cool on wire racks for 10 minutes before serving.

♥ **PER SERVING** Calories: 181.75 | Fat: 6.06 g | Saturated fat: 0.66 g | Sodium: 165.51 mg | Cholesterol: 18.44 mg

Pumpkin Bread

This spicy and velvety bread has the best aroma while it's baking, and it tastes even better.

INGREDIENTS | **YIELDS 1 LOAF: 12 SERVINGS**

½ cup brown sugar

¼ cup sugar

¼ cup canola oil

1 egg

2 egg whites

2 teaspoons vanilla

1 cup canned solid-pack no-salt pumpkin

1¼ cups all-purpose flour

½ cup whole-wheat flour

1 teaspoon baking powder

½ teaspoon baking soda

1 teaspoon cinnamon, divided

¼ teaspoon nutmeg

¼ teaspoon cardamom

2 tablespoons sugar

1. Preheat the oven to 350°F. Spray a 9" × 5" loaf pan with nonstick cooking spray containing flour; set aside.

2. In a large bowl, combine brown sugar, ¼ cup sugar, canola oil, egg, egg whites, and vanilla; beat until combined. Add pumpkin; beat until smooth.

3. Sift together flour, whole-wheat flour, baking powder, baking soda, ½ teaspoon cinnamon, nutmeg, and cardamom. Add to pumpkin mixture; beat until smooth. Spoon batter into prepared pan.

4. In a small bowl, combine 2 tablespoons sugar and ½ teaspoon cinnamon; mix well. Sprinkle over batter.

5. Bake for 60–70 minutes, or until bread is set and toothpick inserted in center comes out clean. Remove from pan and let cool on wire rack.

♥ **PER SERVING** Calories: 178.02 | Fat: 5.63 g | Saturated fat: 0.64 g | Sodium: 108.61 mg | Cholesterol: 35.25 mg

Savory Zucchini Muffins

Serve these flavorful muffins with grilled fish or chicken along with a spinach salad for a nice dinner.

INGREDIENTS | YIELDS 12 MUFFINS

1 tablespoon olive oil

⅓ cup finely chopped onion

4 cloves garlic, minced

¼ cup canola oil

1 cup buttermilk

½ cup egg substitute

1 cup grated zucchini, drained

1¼ cups all-purpose flour

1 cup whole-wheat flour

1 teaspoon baking powder

½ teaspoon baking soda

1 tablespoon fresh chopped rosemary

¼ cup minced flat-leaf parsley

¼ cup grated Parmesan cheese

¼ teaspoon pepper

1. Preheat the oven to 375°F. Line 12 muffin cups with paper liners; set aside.

2. In a small saucepan, combine olive oil, onion, and garlic; cook and stir until tender, about 6 minutes. Remove from heat and place in a large mixing bowl; cool for 30 minutes.

3. Stir in canola oil, buttermilk, egg substitute, and zucchini; mix well. Then add flour, whole-wheat flour, baking powder, baking soda, rosemary, and parsley; mix until dry ingredients are moistened. Stir in cheese and pepper.

4. Fill prepared muffin cups ¾ full. Bake for 20–25 minutes, or until muffins are golden-brown and set. Remove from cups, and serve immediately.

♥ **PER SERVING** Calories: 153.97 | Fat: 7.08 g | Saturated fat: 1.07 g | Sodium: 156.44 mg | Cholesterol: 2.75 mg

Vegetables in Breads

When using vegetables in breads, especially grated vegetables, be sure to drain them well before adding to the batter. Some vegetables, especially zucchini and tomatoes, can add significant amounts of water to the batter and may throw off the proportion of flour to liquid. Follow the recipe carefully.

Whole-Wheat Cinnamon Platters

These crisp and flat rolls are a perfect treat for a special occasion, like Christmas morning or Mother's Day.

INGREDIENTS | YIELDS 18 PLATTERS

1 cup whole-wheat flour

1 (¼-ounce) package instant-blend dry yeast

1¼–1¾ cups all-purpose flour

¼ teaspoon salt

1 teaspoon cinnamon

⅛ teaspoon cardamom

2 tablespoons honey

¼ cup orange juice

½ cup water

1 egg

1 cup dried currants

1 cup sugar

1 cup finely chopped walnuts

2 teaspoons cinnamon

1. In a large bowl, combine whole-wheat flour, yeast, ½ cup all-purpose flour, salt, 1 teaspoon cinnamon, and cardamom; mix well.

2. In a small saucepan, combine honey, orange juice, and water; heat until very warm. Add to flour mixture; beat for 2 minutes.

3. Add egg and beat for 1 minute. Stir in enough remaining all-purpose flour to form a stiff batter. Stir in currants; cover, and let rise for 1 hour.

4. Stir down dough. Line cookie sheets with parchment paper or Silpat liners.

5. On a plate, combine sugar, walnuts, and 2 teaspoons cinnamon; mix well. Drop dough by spoonfuls into sugar mixture; toss to coat. Place on prepared cookie sheets; flatten to ⅛" thick circles.

6. Preheat oven to 400°F. Bake pastries for 13–16 minutes, or until light golden-brown and caramelized. Let cool on cookie sheets for 3 minutes, then remove to wire rack to cool.

♥ **PER SERVING** Calories: 189.56 | Fat: 5.30 g | Saturated fat: 0.77 g | Sodium: 42.47 mg | Cholesterol: 13.44 mg

Whole-Grain Oatmeal Bread

This hearty bread is delicious toasted and spread with whipped honey or jam.

INGREDIENTS | YIELDS 2 LOAVES; 32 SERVINGS

1 cup warm water

2 (¼-ounce) packages active dry yeast

¼ cup honey

1 cup skim milk

1 cup oatmeal

1 teaspoon salt

3 tablespoons canola oil

1 egg

1½ cups whole-wheat flour

½ cup medium rye flour

¼ cup ground flaxseed

3–4 cups bread flour

2 tablespoons butter

Rolls or Bread?

Any yeast bread mixture can be made into rolls. Just divide the dough into 2" balls and roll between your hands to smooth. Place on greased cookie sheets about 4" apart. Cover and let rise for 30–40 minutes. Then bake at 375°F for 15–25 minutes, until deep golden-brown. Let cool on wire racks. Freeze if not using within 1 day.

1. In a small bowl, combine water and yeast; let stand until bubbly, about 5 minutes.

2. In a medium saucepan, combine honey, milk, oatmeal, salt, and canola oil; heat just until very warm (about 120°F). Remove from heat; beat in egg.

3. Combine in a large bowl with whole-wheat flour, rye flour, flaxseed, and 1 cup bread flour. Add yeast mixture; beat for 1 minute. Cover, and let rise for 30 minutes.

4. Gradually stir in enough remaining bread flour to make a firm dough. Turn onto floured surface; knead until dough is elastic, about 10 minutes. Place in a greased bowl, turning to grease top. Cover, and let rise for 1 hour.

5. Punch down dough; divide in half, and form into loaves. Place in two greased 9" × 5" loaf pans; cover, and let rise for 30 minutes.

6. Bake in a preheated 350°F oven for 25–30 minutes, or until golden-brown. Brush with butter, then remove to wire racks to cool.

♥ **PER SERVING** Calories: 136.74 | Fat: 3.46 g | Saturated fat: 0.77 g | Sodium: 85.39 mg | Cholesterol: 8.67 mg

Oat-Bran Dinner Rolls

These excellent rolls are light yet hearty, with a wonderful flavor and a bit of crunch.

INGREDIENTS | YIELDS 30 ROLLS

1½ cups water

¾ cup quick-cooking oats

½ cup oat bran

¼ cup brown sugar

2 tablespoons butter or plant sterol margarine

1 cup buttermilk

2 (¼-ounce) packages active dry yeast

2–3 cups all-purpose flour, divided

1½ cups whole-wheat flour

½ teaspoon salt

2 tablespoons honey

1 egg white, beaten

2 tablespoons oat bran

1. In a medium saucepan, bring water to a boil over high heat. Add oats, oat bran, brown sugar, and butter; stir until butter melts. Remove from heat and let cool to lukewarm.

2. In a microwave-safe glass cup, place buttermilk. Microwave on medium for 1 minute, or until lukewarm (about 110°F). Sprinkle yeast over milk; stir and let stand for 10 minutes.

3. In a large mixing bowl, combine 1 cup all-purpose flour, whole-wheat flour, and salt. Add honey, cooled oatmeal mixture, and softened yeast mixture; beat until smooth. Gradually add enough remaining all-purpose flour to form a soft dough.

4. Turn onto a lightly floured board and knead until smooth and elastic, about 5–7 minutes. Place in a greased bowl, turning to grease top. Cover, and let rise for 1 hour, or until dough doubles.

5. Punch down dough and divide into thirds; divide each third into 10 pieces. Roll balls between your hands to smooth. Place balls into two 9" round cake pans. Brush with egg white and sprinkle with 2 tablespoons oat bran. Cover, and let rise until doubled, about 45 minutes.

6. Preheat the oven to 375°F. Bake rolls for 15–25 minutes, or until firm to the touch and golden-brown. Remove from pans, and cool on wire racks.

♥ **PER SERVING** Calories: 100.84 | Fat: 1.48 g | Saturated fat: 0.64 g | Sodium: 54.45 mg | Cholesterol: 2.36 mg

Cornmeal-Cranberry Rolls

This is a yeast batter bread, which doesn't require kneading.
These little rolls are delicious warm from the oven.

INGREDIENTS | **YIELDS 18 ROLLS**

½ cup buttermilk

½ cup water

½ cup yellow cornmeal

⅓ cup canola oil

2½–3½ cups all-purpose flour

1 (¼-ounce) package instant-blend dried yeast

½ teaspoon salt

1 egg

2 egg whites

⅓ cup honey

⅔ cup chopped dried cranberries

2 tablespoons butter

Instant-Blend Yeast

When a recipe calls for mixing dry yeast with flour and then adding a warm liquid, you should use instant-blend yeast instead of active dry yeast. It performs exactly the same as active dry yeast, but it hydrates much more quickly, so it will come back to life even when surrounded by other ingredients.

1. In a medium saucepan, combine buttermilk, water, cornmeal, and oil over medium heat. Cook, stirring, until very warm. Remove from heat.

2. In a large bowl, combine 2 cups flour, yeast, and salt; mix well. Add buttermilk mixture along with egg, egg whites, and honey; beat for 2 minutes. Gradually add enough remaining flour until a stiff batter forms. Stir in cranberries. Cover, and let rise until doubled, about 1 hour.

3. Grease 18 muffin cups with nonstick cooking spray. Spoon batter into cups, filling each ⅔ full. Cover, and let rise for 30 minutes.

4. Preheat the oven to 350°F. Bake rolls for 20–30 minutes, or until golden-brown and set. Immediately brush with butter. Remove from pans, and let cool on wire racks.

♥ **PER SERVING** Calories: 194.31 | Fat: 6.20 g | Saturated fat: 1.37 g | Sodium: 113.41 mg | Cholesterol: 16.23 mg

Honey-Wheat Sesame Bread

*Sesame seeds add not only flavor and crunch to these delicious
loaves but fiber and healthy monounsaturated fat as well.*

INGREDIENTS | **YIELDS 2 LOAVES; 32 SERVINGS**

1 cup milk

1 cup water

½ cup honey

3 tablespoons butter

¼ teaspoon salt

1 egg

2 cups whole-wheat flour

2 (¼-ounce) packages instant-blend dry yeast

½ cup sesame seeds

3–4 cups all-purpose flour

1 egg white

2 tablespoons sesame seeds

1. In a medium saucepan, combine milk, water, honey, butter, and salt; heat over medium heat until butter melts. Remove from heat; let stand for 30 minutes, or until just lukewarm. Beat in egg.

2. In a large bowl, combine whole-wheat flour, yeast, and ½ cup sesame seeds; add milk mixture and beat for 1 minute. Gradually stir in enough all-purpose flour to make a firm dough.

3. Turn out onto floured surface; knead, adding additional flour if necessary, until dough is elastic. Place in a greased bowl, turning to grease top; cover, and let rise until doubled, about 1 hour.

4. Grease two 9" × 5" loaf pans with unsalted butter; set aside. Punch down dough and divide into 2 parts. On floured surface, roll or pat to 7" × 12" rectangle. Roll up tightly, starting with 7" side. Place in prepared pans. Brush with egg white, and sprinkle each with 1 tablespoon sesame seeds. Cover with towel, and let rise until doubled, about 30 minutes.

5. Preheat the oven to 350°F. Bake loaves for 35–45 minutes, or until golden-brown. Turn onto wire rack to cool completely.

♥ **PER SERVING** Calories: 131.38 | Fat: 3.02 g | Saturated fat: 1.03 g | Sodium: 34.51 mg | Cholesterol: 9.85 mg

Raisin-Cinnamon Oatmeal Bread

Batter breads are really simple to make because they require less of your time.

INGREDIENTS | **YIELDS 2 LOAVES; 32 SERVINGS**

2 (¼-ounce) packages active dry yeast

½ cup warm water

1¼ cups skim milk

¼ cup brown sugar

¼ cup honey

1 egg

2 egg whites

⅓ cup oat bran

1¼ cups oatmeal

3½–4½ cups all-purpose flour

½ teaspoon salt

2 teaspoons cinnamon

2 cups raisins

2 tablespoons butter, melted

Batter Breads

Batter breads are just breads with less flour, so instead of forming a dough they make a stiff batter that becomes difficult to stir. Because the bread isn't kneaded, and there is more liquid, the texture of the bread will be coarser. These breads are quicker to make and are less intimidating to beginning cooks.

1. In a large bowl, combine yeast and warm water; let stand for 10 minutes.

2. In a small saucepan, combine milk, brown sugar, and honey; heat over low heat until warm. Add to yeast along with egg and egg whites; beat until combined.

3. Add oat bran, oatmeal, and 1 cup all-purpose flour; beat for 1 minute. Let stand, covered, for 30 minutes. Then stir in salt, cinnamon, raisins, and enough all-purpose flour to form a stiff batter; beat for 2 minutes.

4. Spray two 9" × 5" loaf pans with nonstick cooking spray. Divide batter among pans, smoothing tops. Cover, and let rise for 45 minutes, until batter is doubled.

5. Preheat the oven to 375°F. Bake bread for 30–40 minutes, or until bread is firm and golden-brown. Remove from pans and brush tops with melted butter; let cool on wire racks.

♥ **PER SERVING** Calories: 138.98 | Fat: 1.60 g | Saturated fat: 0.63 g | Sodium: 54.50 mg | Cholesterol: 8.71 g

Sunflower Rye Bread

*Forming the dough into a round and baking it on a cookie sheet makes
a rustic loaf that is crustier than bread baked in a loaf pan.*

INGREDIENTS | **YIELDS 1 LOAF; 16
SERVINGS**

½ cup lukewarm water
1 (¼-ounce) package active dry yeast
⅔ cup skim milk
¼ cup honey
½ teaspoon salt
2 tablespoons canola oil
1 egg, beaten, divided
1 cup medium rye flour
½ cup whole-wheat flour
2–3 cups bread flour
1 cup hulled unsalted sunflower seeds

1. In a small bowl, combine water and yeast; let stand until bubbly, about 5 minutes.

2. In a microwave-safe glass bowl, combine milk, honey, salt, and canola oil; heat on 30 percent power until warm, about 30-40 seconds. Pour into a large bowl.

3. Remove 1 tablespoon egg and refrigerate for glaze. Add remaining egg to milk mixture along with yeast mixture and rye flour; beat for 1 minute. Add whole-wheat flour and 1 cup bread flour; beat for 1 minute.

4. Gradually stir in enough remaining bread flour to form a firm dough. On a lightly floured surface, knead in sunflower seeds. Knead bread until smooth and elastic, about 10 minutes. Place in a greased bowl, turning to grease top. Cover, and let rise for 1 hour.

5. Punch down dough, and let rest for 10 minutes. On floured surface, shape dough into an 8" round. Spray a cookie sheet with nonstick cooking spray; place dough on sheet. Brush with reserved egg; cover, and let rise for 30 minutes.

6. Preheat the oven to 400°F. Bake for 35–45 minutes or until dark golden-brown. Let cool on a wire rack.

♥ **PER SERVING** Calories: 199.73 | Fat: 6.57 g | Saturated fat: 0.73 g | Sodium: 83.83 mg | Cholesterol: 13.42 mg

Whole-Grain Pizza Crust

*Make a couple of batches of this crust, prebake, and store in the
freezer to make your own homemade pizzas in a flash.*

INGREDIENTS | **YIELDS 2 CRUSTS; 12 SERVINGS**

1 cup warm water

2 (¼-ounce) packages active dry yeast

½ cup skim milk

2 tablespoons honey

2 tablespoons olive oil

½ teaspoon salt

1½ cups whole-wheat flour

1 cup cornmeal

1½–2½ cups bread flour

Freezing Pizza Dough

To freeze pizza dough, bake it for 10 minutes until the crust is set but not browned. Let cool completely, then place in heavy-duty food storage freezer bags, seal, label, and freeze for up to 3 months. To use, you can top the crust right from the freezer and bake as recipe directs, adding 5–10 minutes to the baking time.

1. In a large bowl, combine water and yeast; let stand for 10 minutes until bubbly. Add milk, honey, olive oil, and salt; mix well. Stir in whole-wheat flour, cornmeal, and ½ cup bread flour; beat for 1 minute.

2. Stir in enough bread flour to make a firm dough. Turn onto floured surface; knead for 10 minutes. Place dough in a greased bowl, turning to grease top. Cover, and let rise for 1 hour.

3. Turn dough onto floured work surface; let rest for 10 minutes.

4. Spray two 12" round pizza pans with nonstick cooking spray; sprinkle with some cornmeal. Divide dough in half and roll to 12" circles. Place on pizza pans; press to edges if necessary. Let stand for 10 minutes.

5. Preheat oven to 400°F. Bake crusts for 10 minutes, or until set. Remove from oven, add toppings, return to oven, and bake as pizza recipe directs.

♥ **PER SERVING** Calories: 213.01 | Fat: 3.17 g | Saturated fat: 0.46 g | Sodium: 104.52 mg | Cholesterol: 0.20 mg

Light Whole-Grain Bread

This hearty, crunchy loaf is packed full of flavor, nutrition, and fiber.

INGREDIENTS | YIELDS 2 LOAVES; 32 SERVINGS

1 cup lukewarm water
2 (¼-ounce) packages active dry yeast
1½ cups buttermilk
½ cup orange juice
½ teaspoon salt
⅓ cup honey
3 tablespoons canola oil
1 egg
2 cups whole-wheat flour
½ cup oat bran
½ cup cracked wheat
3½–4½ cups bread flour
½ teaspoon baking soda
2 tablespoons butter

1. In a large bowl, combine water and yeast; mix well. Let stand for 10 minutes. Add buttermilk, orange juice, salt, honey, oil, and egg; beat well.

2. Add 1 cup whole-wheat flour, oat bran, cracked wheat, 1 cup bread flour, and baking soda; beat for 1 minute. Let bread stand for 30 minutes.

3. Gradually add enough remaining whole-wheat flour and bread flour to form a firm dough. Turn onto floured surface; knead for 10 minutes. Place dough in greased bowl, turning to grease top. Cover, and let rise for 1 hour.

4. Turn dough onto floured work surface; let rest for 10 minutes.

5. Grease two 9" × 5" loaf pans with unsalted butter; set aside. Punch down dough and divide into 2 parts. On floured surface, roll or pat to 7" × 12" rectangle. Roll up tightly, starting with 7" side. Place in prepared pans.

6. Cover with towel; let rise until doubled, about 30 minutes.

7. Preheat the oven to 350°F. Bake loaves for 35–45 minutes, or until golden brown. Brush each loaf with butter; turn onto wire rack to cool completely.

♥ **PER SERVING** Calories: 137.87 | Fat: 2.75 g | Saturated fat: 0.74 g | Sodium: 76.58 mg | Cholesterol: 8.98 mg

Whole-Grain Ciabatta

Ciabatta means "slipper" in Italian. The loaves are fairly flat and oblong, with large air holes and a nice crust.

INGREDIENTS | YIELDS 2 LOAVES; 8 SERVINGS

1 cup lukewarm water

1 (¼-ounce) package active dry yeast

⅓ cup milk

2 tablespoons olive oil

¾ cup whole-wheat flour

½ cup oat bran

2–2½ cups bread flour

½ teaspoon salt

2 tablespoons cornmeal

Creating Steam When Baking Bread

Adding steam to the oven when baking bread makes a crisper, thicker crust. There are several ways to do this. You can place a pan with some water in it on the rack below the bread. You can also spritz the loaves with water a few times while the bread is baking. The steam helps keep the bread softer longer, so the crust develops more slowly.

1. In a large bowl, combine water and yeast; stir and let stand for 10 minutes. When yeast is bubbly, add milk, olive oil, whole-wheat flour, oat bran, ½ cup bread flour, and salt; beat for 2 minutes. Cover, and let stand at room temperature for 1 hour.

2. Add enough remaining bread flour to make a soft dough; beat for 1 minute. Cover, and let rise for 1 hour.

3. Remove dough to lightly floured surface (dough will be soft and sticky). Grease two 4" × 10" shapes on a large cookie sheet and sprinkle with cornmeal. Divide dough in half and shape into two 3" × 9" rectangles on the greased areas of the cookie sheet. Let rise for 30 minutes.

4. Preheat the oven to 400°F. Place a 9" pan filled with ½" of water on bottom rack. Bake bread on middle rack for 20–30 minutes, or until loaves are light golden-brown and sound hollow when tapped with fingers. Cool on wire rack.

♥ **PER SERVING** Calories: 212.26 | Fat: 4.62 g | Saturated fat: 0.68 g | Sodium: 152.68 mg | Cholesterol: 0.20 mg

Cornmeal Focaccia

Focaccia dough is not kneaded; this makes the air holes large and texture of the finished bread coarse.

INGREDIENTS | YIELDS 2 LOAVES: 12 SERVINGS

1½–2½ cups all-purpose flour

1 (¼-ounce) package instant-blend dry yeast

1 cup water

1 tablespoon honey

4 tablespoons olive oil, divided

½ teaspoon salt

1 tablespoon chopped fresh rosemary

2 teaspoons chopped fresh oregano leaves

½ cup cornmeal

½ cup masa harina (corn flour)

2 tablespoons cornmeal

¼ cup grated Romano or Cotija cheese

1. In a large bowl, combine 1 cup flour and yeast; mix well.

2. In a microwave-safe glass measuring cup, combine water, honey, 2 tablespoons olive oil, and salt; microwave on 50-percent power for 1 minute, or until mixture is very warm.

3. Add to flour mixture; beat for 2 minutes. Stir in rosemary, oregano, ½ cup cornmeal, and masa harina; beat for 1 minute. Add enough remaining all-purpose flour to make a soft dough. Cover, and let rise for 30 minutes.

4. Divide dough in half. Grease two 12" round pizza pans with unsalted butter and sprinkle with 2 tablespoons cornmeal.

5. Divide dough into 2 parts; press into prepared pans. Push your fingertips into dough to make dimples. Drizzle remaining olive oil over the dough; sprinkle with cheese. Let stand for 20 minutes.

6. Preheat the oven to 425°F. Bake bread for 13–18 minutes, or until deep golden-brown. Cool on wire racks.

♥ **PER SERVING** Calories: 182.86 | Fat: 6.29 g | Saturated fat: 1.50 g | Sodium: 154.62 mg | Cholesterol: 4.91 mg

Three-Grain French Bread

Yogurt and orange juice add a bit of sourdough texture and flavor to this easy and delicious loaf.

INGREDIENTS | **YIELDS 2 LOAVES; 16 SERVINGS**

¾ cup warm water

2 (¼-ounce) packages active dry yeast

1 tablespoon sugar

¼ cup orange juice

1 cup plain yogurt

2 tablespoons lemon juice

1 egg

⅓ cup oat bran

½ teaspoon salt

1½ cups whole-wheat flour

3–3½ cups bread flour

1 tablespoon cornmeal

Storing French Bread

Homemade French bread will not last very long after it's baked. Within two days of baking the bread, slice into 1" slices and flash freeze on a cookie sheet. When bread is frozen, pack into hard-sided containers, label, seal, and freeze up to 3 months. To use, spread with olive oil and toast right out of the freezer.

1. In a large bowl, combine water, yeast, and sugar; stir, and let stand for 10 minutes. Add orange juice, yogurt, lemon juice, and egg; beat for 1 minute. Add oat bran, salt, whole-wheat flour, and 1 cup bread flour; beat. Cover for 1 hour.

2. Gradually add enough remaining bread flour to form a firm dough. Turn onto floured surface; knead for 10 minutes, until smooth and elastic. Place in greased bowl, turning to grease top. Cover, and let rise for 1 hour.

3. Punch down dough; let rest for 10 minutes.

4. With nonstick cooking spray, spray two 14" × 4" rectangles on a cookie sheet; sprinkle with cornmeal. Divide dough in half; roll each half to a 14" × 6" rectangle. Roll up tightly, starting at longer side. Pinch edges and ends to seal; place, seam-side down, on prepared cookie sheet. Cover, and let rise for 30 minutes, or until doubled.

5. Preheat the oven to 375°F. Slash bread in shallow cuts several times, cutting across the loaves, using a sharp knife. Bake for 30–40 minutes, or until loaves are golden-brown and sound hollow when tapped with fingers. Let cool on wire rack.

♥ **PER SERVING** Calories: 158.22 | Fat: 1.61 g | Saturated fat: 0.53 g | Sodium: 85.22 mg | Cholesterol: 15.06 mg

Hearty-Grain French Bread

Cottage cheese, sour cream, and orange juice add a nice tang to this hearty French bread.

INGREDIENTS | **YIELDS 2 LOAVES; 32 SERVINGS**

1 cup quick-cooking oats

1 cup water

½ cup cottage cheese

½ cup low-fat sour cream

2 tablespoons orange juice

½ teaspoon salt

2 cups bread flour

2 (¼-ounce) packages instant-blend dry yeast

¼ cup oat bran

2–3 cups whole-wheat flour

2 tablespoons cornmeal

1. In a small microwave-safe bowl, combine oats and 1 cup water; microwave on high for 3–4 minutes, until creamy. Let cool for 10 minutes.

2. In a blender or food processor, combine oatmeal mixture and cottage cheese; blend or process until creamy.

3. Place oatmeal mixture in a large bowl; stir in sour cream, orange juice, and salt; mix well. Add bread flour, yeast, and oat bran; beat for 1 minute. Stir in enough whole-wheat flour to form a firm dough.

4. Knead dough on a lightly floured surface until smooth and elastic, about 8 minutes. Place in a greased bowl, turning to grease top. Cover and let rise until doubled, about 1 hour.

5. Punch down dough; place on counter. Cover with bowl; let stand for 10 minutes.

6. Grease two 12" long rectangles on a cookie sheet; sprinkle with cornmeal. Divide dough into 2 balls. Roll each ball into a 12" cylinder; place on cookie sheet. Cover, and let rise until doubled, about 30 minutes.

7. Preheat the oven to 375°F. Spray loaves with some cold water; bake for 30–40 minutes, or until loaves are deep golden-brown and sound hollow when tapped with fingers. Cool on a wire rack.

♥ **PER SERVING** Calories: 94.80 | Fat: 1.23 g | Saturated fat: 0.43 g | Sodium: 53.23 mg | Cholesterol: 1.62 mg

Dark Dinner Rolls

Before serving, place these rolls in a 350°F oven for 5–6 minutes to warm and refresh.

INGREDIENTS | **YIELDS 24 ROLLS**

2 cups milk

2 (¼-ounce) packages active dry yeast

¼ cup honey

½ teaspoon salt

3 tablespoons canola oil

1 egg

2 egg whites

2½ cups whole-wheat flour

1½ cups medium rye flour

2½–3 cups all-purpose flour

3 tablespoons butter, melted

Flour Substitutions

You can usually substitute most flours for others, measure for measure. Rye flour, corn flour (masa harina), whole-wheat flour, and buckwheat flour can be used instead of all-purpose flour and bread flour. If you are substituting a lot of whole-grain flours for regular flour, consider using bread flour to help add enough gluten.

1. In a large saucepan, warm milk over medium heat. Pour out ½ cup into a large mixer bowl; combine with yeast. Let stand for 10 minutes.

2. Add remaining milk, honey, salt, canola oil, egg, and egg whites; beat well. Add whole-wheat and rye flours; beat well. Gradually add enough all-purpose flour to form a soft dough.

3. Turn dough onto floured surface; knead until smooth, about 5–7 minutes. Place dough in greased bowl, turning to grease top. Cover, and let rise for 1 hour, or until doubled.

4. Turn dough out onto a lightly floured surface. Divide dough into fourths, then divide each fourth into 6 pieces. Roll pieces between your hands to form a smooth ball. Place on cookie sheets about 3" apart. Let rise for 30–40 minutes, or until doubled.

5. Preheat the oven to 400°F. Bake for 15–25 minutes, or until golden-brown and set. Remove to wire racks, and brush with melted butter. Let cool.

♥ **PER SERVING** Calories: 165.50 | Fat: 4.05 g | Saturated fat: 1.30 g | Sodium: 76.60 mg | Cholesterol: 13.64 mg

Roasted Garlic Bread

*Whole roasted garlic cloves add incredible flavor and texture to this bread.
Toast it, drizzle with olive oil, and serve with a spaghetti dinner.*

INGREDIENTS | YIELDS 2 LOAVES; 32 SERVINGS

1 recipe Light Whole-Grain Bread (see recipe in this chapter)

2 recipes Roasted Garlic (see Chapter 13)

2 tablespoons butter

1. Prepare bread dough; let rise once. Punch down dough; let rest for 10 minutes.

2. Remove cloves of garlic from papery skins, keeping cloves whole; knead into bread. Divide dough in half and shape into 2 ovals.

3. Grease 2 oval shapes on a cookie sheet; place dough on greased spots. Cover, and let rise for 1 hour, until doubled in size.

4. Preheat the oven to 350°F. Bake for 35–45 minutes, or until golden-brown. Brush each loaf with butter; place on wire rack to cool completely.

♥ **PER SERVING** Calories: 156.26 | Fat: 4.05 g | Saturated fat: 1.28 g | Sodium: 92.19 mg | Cholesterol: 10.88 mg

Easy Bread "Sticks"

*These bread sticks are so simple yet so delicious. Serve them alongside
your favorite soup and salad for a hearty lunch.*

INGREDIENTS | SERVES 4

4 (1-ounce) thinly sliced French bread crusts

Olive oil, as needed

1. Preheat the oven to 350°F.

2. Using an oil mister, lightly spray both sides of each slice of bread with olive oil. Arrange on a baking sheet.

3. Bake for 5–10 minutes. (Baking time will depend on the size and thickness of the crusts and on how crisp you want the bread "sticks.")

♥ **PER SERVING** Calories: 77.06 | Protein: 2.31 g | Fat: 0.22 g | Saturated fat: 0.03 g | Sodium: 24.85 mg | Cholesterol: 0.00 mg

Herbed Provence-Style Flatbread (Fougasse)

Traditional fougasse bread is slashed into a pattern resembling an ear of wheat, much like in this recipe. You'll create a fragrant, flavorful loaf.

INGREDIENTS | SERVES 24

Basic White Bread dough (see recipe in this chapter)

2 tablespoons extra-virgin olive oil

½ teaspoon dried rosemary

¼ teaspoon dried French thyme

¼ teaspoon dried tarragon

¼ teaspoon dried basil

¼ teaspoon dried savory

¼ teaspoon dried fennel seeds

¼ teaspoon dried lavender

⅛ teaspoon dried marjoram

⅛ teaspoon freshly ground black pepper

2 tablespoons grated Parmesan cheese

Spectrum Naturals Extra Virgin Olive Spray Oil

When Using a Bread Stone . . .

If baking Fougasse on a bread stone, skip using the olive oil spray and dust your bread peel and the stone with cornmeal to prevent the flatbreads from sticking.

1. Preheat the oven to 450°F.

2. Remove the prepared Basic White Bread dough from refrigerator and punch it down. Lightly coat your hands with olive oil. Divide dough into 24 equal pieces, shaping each piece into a ball. Set aside to rest for a few minutes.

3. Mix together rosemary, thyme, tarragon, basil, savory, fennel seeds, lavender, marjoram, and pepper. Use a mortar and pestle or spice grinder to process into a coarse meal. Stir in the Parmesan cheese.

4. Using your hands, flatten each ball of dough into irregular shapes to give character to the bread.

5. Spray a baking sheet with the olive oil spray; place dough on sheet. With a pastry scraper, *lame* (a tool used to slit the tops of bread loaves), or X-acto knife (kept specifically for that purpose), cut 3 or 4 lengthwise slashes into the bread. Gently pull apart at the slashes. Cover with a clean towel, and let rest for 10 minutes.

6. Brush lightly with olive oil; sprinkle with herb-Parmesan topping. Bake until golden and crusty, about 15–18 minutes.

♥ **PER SERVING** Calories: 98.79 | Fat: 2.59 g | Saturated fat: 0.42 g | Sodium: 105.16 mg | Cholesterol: 0.33 mg

Banana-Rum Mousse

You can serve this mousse immediately after blending, or place it in goblets or sherbet cups and freeze before serving.

INGREDIENTS | SERVES 4

3 tablespoons rum
2 tablespoons lime juice
2 tablespoons powdered sugar
2 bananas, chopped
1 cup vanilla frozen yogurt
4 sprigs fresh mint, for garnish

1. In a blender or food processor, combine the rum, lime juice, sugar, and bananas; blend or process until smooth.

2. Add the yogurt; blend or process until smooth, scraping down sides once during blending.

3. Spoon into dessert glasses; serve immediately with mint sprigs, or cover and freeze up to 8 hours before serving.

♥ **PER SERVING** Calories: 164.58 | Fat: 2.25 g | Saturated fat: 1.13 g | Sodium: 32.30 mg | Cholesterol: 0.72 mg

Green Grapes with Lemon Sorbet

This simple dish brings out the flavor and juicy sweetness of grapes. If you don't want to use wine, try pear nectar or white grape juice instead.

INGREDIENTS | SERVES 4

2 cups green grapes
2 tablespoons sugar
½ cup sweet white wine
1 teaspoon orange zest
2 cups lemon sorbet

1. Wash grapes; dry, and cut in half.

2. Sprinkle sugar over grapes; let stand for 5 minutes.

3. Add wine; stir gently until sugar dissolves. Sprinkle with orange zest; cover, and refrigerate for 1 hour.

4. When ready to serve, stir; serve over sorbet in sherbet glasses or goblets.

♥ **PER SERVING** Calories: 233.90 | Fat: 1.61 g | Saturated fat: 0.90 g | Sodium: 35.64 mg | Cholesterol: 0.00 mg

Lemon Mousse

Pear nectar is very mild, and it adds a nice bit of sweetness to this tart mousse.

Pasteurized Egg Whites

You can find pasteurized eggs in any grocery store. Be sure to carefully abide by the sell-by and use-by dates that are stamped on the package and usually on each egg. Pasteurized egg whites take longer to whip to peaks than ordinary eggs; just keep beating them until the peaks form. Cream of tartar helps stabilize the foam.

1. In a microwave-safe glass measuring cup, combine gelatin and cold water; let stand for 5 minutes to soften gelatin.

2. Stir in lemon juice, pear nectar, 2 tablespoons sugar, and lemon zest; microwave on high for 1–2 minutes, stirring twice during cooking time, until sugar and gelatin completely dissolve. Let cool for 30 minutes.

3. When gelatin mixture is cool to the touch, blend in yogurt.

4. In a medium bowl, combine egg whites with cream of tartar; beat until soft peaks form. Gradually stir in remaining 2 tablespoons sugar, beating until stiff peaks form.

5. Fold gelatin mixture into egg whites until combined. Pour into serving glasses or goblets; cover, and chill until firm, about 4–6 hours.

♥ **PER SERVING** Calories: 151.27 | Fat: 0.65 g | Saturated fat: 0.40 g | Sodium: 65.70 mg | Cholesterol: 2.27 mg

Blueberry Cloud

This can be made with many other fruits. Chopped strawberries, raspberries (fresh or frozen), and peaches would all be delicious.

INGREDIENTS | SERVES 4

1 (0.25-ounce) envelope unflavored gelatin

¼ cup cold water

¾ cup orange juice

3 tablespoons sugar

1 cup blueberries

1 cup vanilla frozen yogurt

1 cup frozen nonfat whipped topping, thawed

1. In a microwave-safe glass measuring cup, combine gelatin with water; let stand for 5 minutes.

2. Add orange juice and sugar; microwave on high for 1–2 minutes, stirring twice during cooking time, until gelatin and sugar dissolve. Pour into a blender or food processor.

3. Add berries; blend or process until smooth. Let stand until cool, about 20 minutes.

4. Add yogurt; process until smooth. Pour into medium bowl; fold in whipped topping. Spoon into serving dishes; cover, and freeze for at least 4 hours before serving.

♥ **PER SERVING** Calories: 183.28 | Fat: 4.72 g | Saturated fat: 3.37 g | Sodium: 49.08 mg | Cholesterol: 1.10 mg

Peach Melba Parfait

This fresh and easy dessert can be made with many flavor combinations. Try sliced pears with orange yogurt and mandarin orange segments.

INGREDIENTS | SERVES 4

4 ripe peaches, peeled and sliced

1 tablespoon lemon juice

2 tablespoons sugar

1 cup raspberry yogurt

1 pint fresh raspberries

4 sprigs fresh mint

1. In a medium bowl, combine the peaches, lemon juice, and sugar; let stand for 10 minutes. Stir to dissolve sugar.

2. In 4 parfait or wine glasses, place some of the peach mixture. Top with a spoonful of the yogurt, then some fresh raspberries. Repeat layers, ending with raspberries.

3. Cover, and chill for 2–4 hours before serving. Garnish with mint sprig.

♥ **PER SERVING** Calories: 153.23 | Fat: 1.26 g | Saturated fat: 0.43 g | Sodium: 33.57 mg | Cholesterol: 2.27 mg

Strawberry-Rhubarb Parfait

Rhubarb is one of the first vegetables (yes, vegetables!) to start growing in the spring. Combined with strawberries, it has a wonderfully tart and refreshing flavor.

INGREDIENTS | SERVES 6

2 stalks rhubarb, sliced
½ cup apple juice
⅓ cup sugar
1 (10-ounce) package frozen strawberries
3 cups frozen vanilla yogurt

1. In a medium saucepan, combine rhubarb, apple juice, and sugar. Bring to a simmer; reduce heat and simmer for 8–10 minutes, or until rhubarb is soft.

2. Remove pan from heat; immediately stir in frozen strawberries, stirring to break up strawberries. Let stand until cool, about 30 minutes

3. Layer rhubarb mixture and frozen yogurt in parfait glasses or goblets, starting and ending with rhubarb mixture. Cover, and freeze until firm, about 8 hours.

♥ **PER SERVING** Calories: 210.56 | Fat: 4.16 g | Saturated fat: 2.48 g | Sodium: 64.41 mg | Cholesterol: 1.44 mg

Chocolate Mousse Banana Meringue Pie

This luxurious and delicious pie is low-fat, yet full of flavor. You could top it with a dollop of frozen nondairy whipped topping for a garnish if you'd like.

INGREDIENTS | SERVES 8

1 meringue pie shell (see Strawberry-Mango Meringue Pie recipe in this chapter)
3 tablespoons cocoa powder
1 recipe Silken Chocolate Mousse (see recipe in this chapter)
2 bananas, sliced
1 tablespoon lemon juice

1. Follow directions to make Meringue Pie Shell, but also beat cocoa into egg whites along with the sugar. Bake as directed in recipe. Let cool completely.

2. Make mousse as directed; chill in bowl for 4–6 hours, until firm. Slice bananas, sprinkling lemon juice over slices as you work.

3. Layer mousse and sliced bananas in pie shell, beginning and ending with mousse. Cover, and chill for 2–3 hours before serving.

♥ **PER SERVING** Calories: 253.53 | Fat: 9.23 g | Saturated fat: 5.94 g | Sodium: 79.66 mg | Cholesterol: 8.71 mg

Crepes with Poached Pears

You can fill these crepes with anything from strawberries and yogurt to Silken Chocolate Mousse (see recipe in this chapter). Keep a batch in the freezer for last-minute desserts.

INGREDIENTS | SERVES 6

1 egg

½ cup 1% milk

½ cup flour

2 tablespoons sugar

2 tablespoons melted butter, divided

4 pears

¼ cup sugar

2 tablespoons lemon juice

¼ cup pear nectar

½ cup frozen nondairy whipped topping, thawed

1 cup fresh raspberries

2 tablespoons powdered sugar

1. In a blender or food processor, combine egg, milk, flour, sugar, and 1 tablespoon melted butter; blend or process until smooth. Let stand for 15 minutes.

2. Heat a 7" nonstick skillet over medium heat. Brush with melted butter. Using a ¼-cup measure, pour 2 tablespoons batter into the skillet; immediately rotate and tilt skillet to spread batter evenly. Cook over medium heat for 1–2 minutes, or until crepe can be moved.

3. Loosen the edges of crepe and flip; cook for 1 minute on second side, then turn out onto kitchen towels. Stack between layers of waxed or parchment paper when cool.

4. For filling, peel and chop pears; place in medium saucepan with sugar and lemon juice. Pour pear nectar over. Bring to a simmer over medium-high heat; cook, stirring gently, until pears are very tender, about 3–5 minutes.

5. Let pears cool in liquid. When ready to serve, fold pear mixture into whipped topping. Fill crepes with this mixture and place, seam-side down, on serving plates. Garnish with raspberries and sprinkle with powdered sugar.

♥ **PER SERVING** Calories: 185.51 | Fat: 5.93 g | Saturated fat: 3.54 g | Sodium: 62.39 mg | Cholesterol: 46.56 mg

Strawberry-Mango Meringue Pie

Meringue pie shells have absolutely no fat at all, and are the perfect foil for almost any filling.

INGREDIENTS | SERVES 8

1 teaspoon flour
3 egg whites
½ teaspoon cream of tartar
½ cup sugar
1 teaspoon vanilla
1 (8-ounce) package low-fat cream cheese, softened
1 cup mango yogurt
1 cup chopped strawberries
2 mangoes, peeled and chopped

Mangoes

It isn't difficult to prepare a mango; it just takes practice. Hold the mango upright on work surface, then cut down the sides, avoiding the long oval pit in the center. Then hold the halves in your palm and score the fruit in a cross-hatch pattern. Turn the halves inside-out and cut the cubes from the skin.

1. Preheat the oven to 300°F. Spray a 9" pie plate with nonstick cooking spray and dust with 1 teaspoon flour.

2. In a large bowl, combine egg whites and cream of tartar; beat until soft peaks form. Gradually beat in sugar until very stiff peaks form. Beat in vanilla. Spread into prepared pan, building up sides to form a shell.

3. Bake for 50–60 minutes, or until shell is very light golden and dry to the touch. Turn oven off and let stand in oven for 1 hour. Cool completely.

4. For filling, in a medium bowl, beat cream cheese until fluffy. Gradually add yogurt; beat until well combined. Fold in strawberries and mangoes.

5. Spoon into meringue pie shell; cover, and chill for 3–4 hours before serving.

♥ **PER SERVING** Calories: 195.15 | Fat: 5.51 g | Saturated fat: 3.40 g | Sodium: 123.32 mg | Cholesterol: 17.10 mg

Loco Pie Crust

*Yes, mayonnaise in pie crust! The egg and oil in the mayonnaise
make the crust tender, while adding a nice flavor.*

INGREDIENTS | SERVES 8

½ cup plus 1 tablespoon mayonnaise

3 tablespoons buttermilk

1 teaspoon vinegar

1½ cups flour

Freezing Pie Crusts

Prepared pie crusts and most regular recipes are full of fat, and solid shortenings have lots of trans fat. You can make double batches of this recipe and freeze one crust for later use. Keep the waxed paper on the crust and slip into a large freezer bag. Label, seal, and freeze for up to 3 months. Thaw by standing at room temperature for 30 minutes.

1. In a large bowl, combine mayonnaise, buttermilk, and vinegar; mix well. Add flour; stir with a fork to form a ball. You may need to add more buttermilk or more flour to make a workable dough.

2. Press dough into a ball; wrap in plastic wrap, and refrigerate for 1 hour.

3. When ready to bake, preheat the oven to 400°F. Roll out dough between 2 sheets of waxed paper. Remove top sheet and place crust in 9" pie pan. Carefully ease off top sheet of paper, then ease crust into pan; press to bottom and sides. Fold edges under and flute.

4. Either use as recipe directs, or bake for 5 minutes, then press crust down with fork, if necessary. Bake for 5–8 minutes longer, or until crust is light golden-brown.

♥ **PER SERVING** Calories: 171.83 | Fat: 7.35 g | Saturated fat: 1.18 g | Sodium: 65.46 mg | Cholesterol: 0.68 mg

Lite Creamy Cheesecake

The secret to this cheesecake is to make sure that the cottage cheese is completely smooth before proceeding with the recipe.

INGREDIENTS | SERVES 12

1½ cups crushed gingersnap crumbs

⅓ cup finely chopped walnuts

2 tablespoons butter or margarine, melted

2 tablespoons orange juice

1½ cups nonfat cottage cheese

1 cup sugar

¼ cup orange juice

2 tablespoons lemon juice

1 (8-ounce) package light cream cheese, softened

1 (3-ounce) package nonfat cream cheese, softened

1 cup nonfat sour cream

1 egg

3 egg whites

¼ cup cornstarch

1 tablespoon vanilla

1. Preheat the oven to 350°F.

2. In a medium bowl, combine gingersnap crumbs, walnuts, butter, and 2 tablespoons orange juice; mix until even. Press into bottom and up sides of 9" springform pan; set aside in refrigerator.

3. In a blender or food processor, combine cottage cheese, sugar, ¼ cup orange juice, and lemon juice; blend or process until very smooth. Scrape down sides; blend or process again.

4. In a large mixing bowl, combine both packages of cream cheese; beat until smooth. Add sour cream; beat again until smooth. Add egg and beat well; add cottage cheese mixture and beat well. Stir in egg whites, cornstarch, and vanilla; beat until smooth.

5. Pour into crust. Bake for 50–60 minutes, or until cheesecake is set around edges but still soft in center. Remove from oven and place on wire rack; let cool for 1 hour. Cover and refrigerate until cold, at least 4 hours.

♥ **PER SERVING** Calories: 254.77 | Fat: 9.11 g | Saturated fat: 4.07 g | Sodium: 206.98 mg | Cholesterol: 37.05 mg

Silken Chocolate Mousse

This velvety-smooth and rich mousse has the best texture. Top it with some fresh raspberries for the perfect finish.

INGREDIENTS | SERVES 6

2 (1-ounce) squares unsweetened chocolate

2 tablespoons butter

½ cup sugar

1 teaspoon vanilla

½ cup satin or silken soft tofu

1 cup chocolate frozen yogurt

1 cup frozen nondairy whipped topping, thawed

Silken Tofu

Make sure that you use silken tofu in this or any other mousse or pudding recipe. Do not use the block type that floats in water. Silken tofu may be packaged in aseptic packaging and stocked on the grocery shelves, not the dairy aisle. All tofu is made of the same ingredients; it's processed differently to make the different types.

1. Chop chocolate; place in a small microwave-safe bowl with butter. Microwave on medium for 2–4 minutes, stirring twice during cooking time, until chocolate is melted and mixture is smooth. Stir in sugar until dissolved.

2. In a blender or food processor, place chocolate mixture; add vanilla and tofu; blend or process until smooth. If necessary, let cool for 10–15 minutes, or until lukewarm.

3. Add frozen yogurt; blend or process until smooth. Add whipped topping; blend or process until just mixed.

4. Spoon into serving glasses; cover, and chill for 4–6 hours before serving.

♥ **PER SERVING** Calories: 219.73 | Fat: 12.12 g | Saturated fat: 7.86 g | Sodium: 78.14 mg | Cholesterol: 11.62 mg

Peach Granita with Raspberry Coulis

Granita is made by freezing a liquid and periodically stirring it, so it freezes in larger crystals and has a grainy texture.

INGREDIENTS | SERVES 8

½ cup orange juice

¼ plus ⅓ cup sugar, divided

2 peaches, peeled and sliced

1½ cups peach nectar

1 teaspoon vanilla

¼ cup lemon juice, divided

1 tablespoon corn syrup

1 (10-ounce) package frozen raspberries, thawed

1 teaspoon vanilla

2 tablespoons raspberry liqueur

1. In a small pan, combine orange juice and ⅓ cup sugar; bring to a simmer, stirring frequently, until sugar dissolves.

2. In a blender or food processor, combine peach slices, nectar, vanilla, 2 tablespoons lemon juice, and corn syrup; blend or process until smooth. Add orange juice mixture; blend or process again until smooth.

3. Pour mixture into a 9" square glass pan. Freeze for 1 hour; remove from freezer and stir. Continue freezing for about 4 hours, stirring every 30 minutes, until a granular frozen texture forms.

4. In a blender or food processor, combine raspberries, ¼ cup sugar, remaining 2 tablespoons lemon juice, 1 teaspoon vanilla, and raspberry liqueur; blend or process until smooth.

5. Stir granita, and spoon into dessert cups or goblets. Pour raspberry coulis over, and serve immediately.

♥ **PER SERVING** Calories: 162.59 | Fat: 0.22 g | Saturated fat: 0.02 g | Sodium: 5.15 mg | Cholesterol: 0.00 mg

Apple-Date Turnovers

Traditionally, turnovers are made of puff pastry, which is loaded with saturated fat.
Using filo dough reduces the fat and increases the crispness.

INGREDIENTS | YIELDS 12 TURNOVERS

2 Granny Smith apples, peeled and chopped

½ cup finely chopped dates

1 teaspoon lemon juice

1 tablespoon flour

3 tablespoons brown sugar

1½ teaspoons cinnamon, divided

8 (14" × 18") sheets frozen filo dough, thawed

½ cup finely chopped walnuts

5 tablespoons sugar, divided

⅓ cup butter or margarine, melted

Filo Dough

Filo dough, also called fillo dough or phyllo dough, is paper-thin layers of dough used in Greek cooking. You can find it in the frozen foods aisle of the grocery store. Carefully follow the instructions for thawing and using on the box. The dough dries out in minutes, so be sure to keep it covered with a damp (not wet) towel while you're working with it.

1. In a medium bowl, combine apples, dates, lemon juice, flour, brown sugar, and 1 teaspoon cinnamon; mix well, and set aside.

2. Place thawed filo dough on work surface; cover with a damp kitchen towel to prevent drying. Work with one sheet at a time.

3. In a small bowl, combine walnuts and 3 tablespoons sugar.

4. Lay one filo sheet on work surface; brush with butter. Sprinkle with 2 tablespoons of walnut mixture. Place another filo sheet on top; brush with butter, and sprinkle with 1 tablespoon of walnut mixture. Cut into three 4¾" × 18" strips.

5. Place 2 tablespoons of apple filling at one end of dough strips. Fold a corner of dough over filling so edges match; continue folding dough as you would fold a flag. Place on ungreased cookie sheets; brush with more butter. Repeat process with remaining strips. Preheat the oven to 375°F.

6. In a small bowl, combine remaining 2 tablespoons sugar and ½ teaspoon cinnamon; mix well. Sprinkle over turnovers.

7. Bake for 20–30 minutes, or until pastries are golden-brown and crisp. Remove to wire racks to cool.

♥ **PER SERVING** Calories: 182.02 | Fat: 9.01 g | Saturated fat: 3.61 g | Sodium: 99.11 mg | Cholesterol: 13.56 mg

Lemon Floating Island

Floating island refers to the poached egg-white mixture that "floats" on the lemon mousse. This is a low-fat version of lemon meringue pie. Yum!

INGREDIENTS | SERVES 4

2 cups milk

6 egg whites

2 tablespoons lemon juice

½ cup sugar

Pinch salt

6 tablespoons crushed hard lemon candies, divided

1 recipe Lemon Mousse (see recipe in this chapter)

1. Preheat the oven to 275°F.

2. In a large skillet, add milk and bring to a simmer over medium heat; reduce heat to low.

3. In a large bowl, combine egg whites and lemon juice; beat until foamy. Gradually add sugar and salt; beat until very stiff peaks form. Fold in 3 tablespoons of crushed candies.

4. With a large spoon, scoop out about ¼ cup of egg white mixture; gently place in simmering milk. Poach for 2 minutes; carefully turn each meringue and poach another 2 minutes. Remove from heat; drain briefly on kitchen towel, and place on Silpat-lined cookie sheets.

5. Bake for 12–16 minutes, or until they puff slightly and start to turn light golden-brown. Remove; refrigerate, uncovered, for 1–2 hours before serving.

6. When you prepare the Lemon Mousse, spoon into individual custard cups; chill until firm. Top each with a poached meringue and sprinkle with remaining 3 tablespoons crushed candies; serve immediately.

♥ **PER SERVING** Calories: 295.74 | Fat: 0.80 g | Saturated fat: 0.45 g | Sodium: 190.06 mg | Cholesterol: 2.65 mg

Whole-Wheat Chocolate Chip Cookies

Fill your cookie jar with these excellent cookies! They're high in fiber yet studded with delicious dark-chocolate nuggets.

INGREDIENTS | YIELDS 18 COOKIES

¼ cup butter or plant sterol margarine, softened

1½ cups brown sugar

½ cup applesauce

1 tablespoon vanilla

1 egg

2 egg whites

2½ cups whole-wheat pastry flour

½ cup ground oatmeal

1 teaspoon baking soda

¼ teaspoon salt

2 cups special dark chocolate chips

1 cup chopped hazelnuts

1. Preheat the oven to 375°F. Line cookie sheets with parchment paper or Silpat silicone liners; set aside.

2. In a large bowl, combine butter, brown sugar, and applesauce; beat well until smooth. Add vanilla, egg, and egg whites; beat until combined.

3. Add flour, oatmeal, baking soda, and salt; mix until a dough forms. Fold in chocolate chips and hazelnuts.

4. Drop dough by rounded teaspoons onto prepared cookie sheets. Bake for 7–10 minutes, or until cookies are light golden-brown and set. Let cool for 5 minutes before removing from cookie sheet to wire rack to cool.

♥ **PER SERVING** Calories: 114.86 | Fat: 4.89 g | Saturated fat: 2.04 g | Sodium: 26.49 mg | Cholesterol: 6.95 mg

Whole-Wheat Pastry Flour

Whole-wheat pastry flour isn't the same as whole-wheat flour; it's slightly lighter and finer for baking. You can find it in specialty stores and online. You can substitute plain whole-wheat flour if you can't find the pastry flour, but use 2 tablespoons less per cup. With plain flour, the product will be denser, with a stronger flavor.

Oatmeal Brownies

*Ground oatmeal, prune purée, and finely chopped dates add great
chewy texture (and fiber) to these easy brownies.*

INGREDIENTS | **YIELDS 16 BROWNIES**

¼ cup prune purée

¼ cup finely chopped dates

½ cup all-purpose flour

½ cup ground oatmeal

½ cup cocoa powder

½ teaspoon baking soda

½ cup brown sugar

¼ cup sugar

1 egg

1 egg white

¼ cup chocolate yogurt

2 teaspoons vanilla

2 tablespoons butter or plant sterol
margarine, melted

½ cup dark chocolate chips

1. Preheat the oven to 350°F. Spray an 8" square baking
   pan with nonstick cooking spray containing flour; set
   aside.

2. In a small bowl, combine prune purée and dates; mix
   well and set aside.

3. In a large bowl, combine flour, oatmeal, cocoa, baking
   soda, brown sugar, and sugar; mix well.

4. Add egg, egg white, yogurt, vanilla, and butter to prune
   mixture; mix well. Add to flour mixture; stir just until
   blended. Spoon into prepared pan; smooth top.

5. Bake for 22–30 minutes, or until edges are set but
   center is still slightly soft. Remove from oven, and place
   on wire rack.

6. In a microwave-safe bowl, place chocolate chips.
   Microwave on 50 percent power for 1 minute; remove
   and stir. Microwave for 30 seconds longer, then stir. If
   necessary, repeat microwave process until chips are
   melted. Pour over warm brownies; gently spread to
   cover. Let cool completely, and cut into bars.

♥ **PER SERVING** Calories: 153.83 | Fat: 4.88 g | Saturated fat:
2.63 g | Sodium: 63.58 mg | Cholesterol: 17.39 mg

Butterscotch Meringues

The candies have to be very finely crushed for best results. This simple little cookie is loaded with flavor.

INGREDIENTS | YIELDS 30 COOKIES

3 egg whites
Pinch of salt
¼ teaspoon cream of tartar
⅔ cup sugar
2 tablespoons brown sugar
10 round hard butterscotch candies, finely crushed

1. Preheat the oven to 250°F.

2. In a large bowl, beat egg whites with salt and cream of tartar until foamy. Gradually beat in sugar and brown sugar until stiff peaks form and sugar is dissolved. Fold in the finely crushed candies.

3. Drop by teaspoonfuls onto a baking sheet lined with aluminum foil or Silpat liners.

4. Bake for 50–60 minutes, or until meringues are set and crisp and very light golden-brown. Cool on cookie sheets for 3 minutes, then carefully peel cookies off foil, and place on wire racks to cool.

♥ **PER SERVING** Calories: 29.39 | Fat: 0.06 g | Saturated fat: 0.04 g | Sodium: 17.97 mg | Cholesterol: 0.16 mg

Tofu, Oil, and Vinegar Salad Dressing

This dressing is a blank canvas for you to experiment with. Use your favorite flavors, or try something new!

INGREDIENTS | SERVES 4

1 tablespoon extra-virgin olive oil
2 tablespoons silken tofu
1 tablespoon vinegar
1 teaspoon ground mustard
Choice of herbs, spices, and freshly ground black pepper (optional)

Place all the ingredients in a small bowl and whisk to combine. Pour over your choice of prepared salad greens and vegetables.

♥ **PER SERVING** Calories: 35.82 | Fat: 3.69 g | Saturated fat: 0.50 g | Sodium: 0.61 mg | Cholesterol: 0.00 mg

Saffron Vinaigrette

Saffron is a spice taken from the saffron crocus, and its dried stigmas are used in cooking. It's flavor is hay-like and sweet, and it adds a yellow color to foods.

INGREDIENTS | SERVES 16

1 cup dry white wine

1 cup rice wine or white wine vinegar

1 tablespoon chopped shallots

3 peppercorns, crushed

½ teaspoon dried thyme

¼ teaspoon saffron

½ cup extra-virgin olive oil

½ tablespoon honey

1. In a saucepan over medium-low heat, add the wine, vinegar, shallots, peppercorns, thyme, and saffron; slowly reduce by half to yield ½ cup of liquid.

2. Strain the mixture through a fine-mesh sieve.

3. Whisk in the olive oil and honey. Use immediately to wilt lettuce, or chill until ready to serve.

♥ **PER SERVING** Calories: 74.24 | Fat: 6.75 g | Saturated fat: 0.91 g | Sodium: 0.99 mg | Cholesterol: 0.00 mg

Pear Salad with Fat-Free Raspberry Vinaigrette

The tang of the raspberry vinaigrette pairs nicely with the sweet pears. Walnuts and blue cheese add to the elegant flavor combination.

INGREDIENTS | SERVES 4

2 tablespoons Cascadian Farm frozen Organic Raspberry Juice Concentrate

2 tablespoons water

1 tablespoon white wine vinegar

1 tablespoon plain nonfat yogurt

⅛ teaspoon freshly ground black or white pepper

4 cups mixed salad greens (such as iceberg lettuce, green leaf lettuce, romaine, and radicchio), torn into bite-sized pieces

2 medium-size Bartlett pears, peeled, sliced, and diced

¼ cup chopped walnuts, toasted

2 ounces blue cheese, crumbled

1. In a small bowl, combine the raspberry juice concentrate, water, white wine vinegar, yogurt, and pepper; whisk well to combine.

2. Toss the salad greens with the vinaigrette. Divide the greens between 4 serving plates. Top with the pears, nuts, and blue cheese. Serve immediately.

♥ **PER SERVING** Calories: 420.79 | Fat: 36.41 g | Saturated fat: 6.79 g | Sodium: 207.48 mg | Cholesterol: 10.71 mg

Thousand Island Dressing

Traditional Thousand Island dressing uses a lot of mayonnaise, and isn't exactly a healthy choice. This healthier version scales down the amount of mayo, but is just as delicious.

INGREDIENTS | SERVES 16

½ cup plain nonfat yogurt

2 tablespoons Hellmann's or Best Foods Real Mayonnaise

2 tablespoons low-salt ketchup

1 tablespoon Cascadian Farm Sweet Relish

1 teaspoon lemon juice

1 teaspoon apple cider vinegar

1 tablespoon finely chopped celery

½ teaspoon granulated sugar or ¼ teaspoon honey

¼ teaspoon celery seed

¼ teaspoon onion powder

¼ teaspoon yellow or Dijon mustard

⅛ teaspoon mustard powder

⅛ teaspoon freshly ground black pepper

1 large hard-boiled egg, minced

1. Add all ingredients to a jar. Cover, and shake well to combine.

2. Refrigerate between uses. Can be stored 3–4 days. To serve, shake well to emulsify.

♥ **PER SERVING** Calories: 31.74 | Fat: 1.90 g | Saturated fat: 0.27 g | Sodium: 70.52 mg | Cholesterol: 14.41 mg

Russian Dressing

This is a healthy version of the classic dressing used on Reuben sandwiches. It's fantastic on salads as well.

INGREDIENTS | SERVES 18

½ cup grapeseed or canola oil

¼ cup red wine or balsamic vinegar (or a combination)

¼ cup water

½ teaspoon Dijon mustard

1 teaspoon garlic powder

1 teaspoon onion powder

¼ teaspoon mustard powder

¼ teaspoon freshly ground black pepper

¼ teaspoon granulated sugar

¼ teaspoon dried basil

¼–½ teaspoon salt-free chili powder

¼–½ teaspoon sweet paprika

2 tablespoons Muir Glen No-Salt-Added Tomato Paste

Pinch dried red pepper flakes

1 tablespoon finely chopped green bell pepper

1. Add all the ingredients to a jar. Cover, and shake well to combine.

2. Refrigerate between uses. To serve, shake well to emulsify.

♥ **PER SERVING** Calories: 61.48 | Fat: 6.27 g | Saturated fat: 0.59 g | Sodium: 78.93 mg | Cholesterol: 0.00 mg

Creamy Russian Dressing

To make a single serving of Creamy Russian Dressing, mix together 1 tablespoon Russian Dressing, 1 teaspoon Hellmann's or Best Foods Real Mayonnaise, and 2 teaspoons plain nonfat yogurt. Nutritional analysis per serving: Calories: 104.96; Protein: 1.51 g; Carbohydrates: 2.72 g; Fat: 9.96 g; Saturated Fat: 1.01 g; Cholesterol: 3.09 mg; Sodium: 119.44 mg.

Candied Walnut Salad with Pomegranate Vinaigrette

This salad makes an elegant first course—serve it at your next dinner party to impress your guests.

INGREDIENTS | SERVES 4

⅛ cup chopped walnuts

2 tablespoons sherry

1 tablespoon granulated sugar

2 tablespoons extra-virgin olive oil

1 tablespoon balsamic vinegar

1 teaspoon pomegranate concentrated juice or molasses

⅛ cup water

¼ teaspoon Dijon mustard

Pinch mustard powder

Pinch freshly ground black pepper

4 cups mixed salad greens, torn into bite-size pieces

1 mango or peach, peeled, pitted, and diced

1 ripe pear, peeled, cored, and diced

1 ripe avocado, peeled, pitted, and sliced

1 ounce blue cheese, crumbled

1. Add the walnuts, sherry, and sugar to a small nonstick sauté pan over high heat. Stir constantly with a wooden spoon until the sherry and sugar caramelize on the walnuts. Set aside to cool.

2. Add the oil, vinegar, pomegranate, water, mustard, mustard powder, and pepper to a jar; shake until smooth and creamy.

3. Toss the salad greens, mango, and pear with the dressing. Divide between 4 serving plates. Arrange the avocado slices evenly around the salads. Top with the crumbled blue cheese and candied walnuts.

♥ **PER SERVING** Calories: 290.46 | Fat: 19.67 g | Saturated fat: 3.67 g | Sodium: 285.13 mg | Cholesterol: 5.32 mg

Instant Fat-Free Salad Dressing

Mix some of your favorite fruit jelly with an equal amount American Spoon Foods jalapeño jelly. Add freeze-dried green onion or shallots and vinegar to taste; thin with a little water, if necessary.

French Dressing

This dressing has an incredible blend of herbs and spices to add some kick to your salads.

INGREDIENTS | SERVES 18

¼ cup water

1 tablespoon freeze-dried shallots or dried minced onion

1 clove garlic, crushed

½ cup extra-virgin olive oil

¼ cup red wine vinegar

¼ teaspoon Dijon mustard

¼ teaspoon mustard powder

¼ teaspoon freshly ground black pepper

2 teaspoons honey

½ teaspoon dried basil

¼ teaspoon dried tarragon

⅛ teaspoon dried rosemary

⅛ teaspoon dried thyme

2 tablespoons Muir Glen Organic No-Salt-Added Tomato Paste

1. Bring the water to a boil. Add the shallots and garlic to a jar; pour the boiling water over them. Cover the jar and let rest at room temperature for 30 minutes to bring out the flavors and reconstitute the shallots. Use a slotted spoon to remove and discard the garlic.

2. Add the remaining ingredients to the jar; cover, and shake well to combine.

3. Refrigerate between uses. To serve, allow 10 minutes for the dressing to come to room temperature and for the olive oil to become liquid again. Shake well to emulsify.

♥ **PER SERVING** Calories: 61.12 | Fat: 6.11 g | Saturated fat: 0.82 g | Sodium: 40.12 mg | Cholesterol: 0.00 mg

APPENDIX A

Resources

Cardiovascular Disease Resources

American Heart Association
www.americanheart.org

American Lung Association
www.lungusa.org

Cardiovascular Risk-Assessment Calculator
http://hp2010.nhlbihin.net/atpiii/calculator.asp

Stanford Prevention Resource Center, Stanford University School of Medicine
http://prevention.stanford.edu

American Diabetes Association
www.diabetes.org

National Cholesterol Education Program
www.nhlbi.nih.gov/about/ncep

NIH ATP3 Cholesterol Guidelines
www.nhlbi.nih.gov/guidelines/cholesterol

Health Organization Resources

American Red Cross
www.redcross.org

Centers for Disease Control and Prevention (CDC)
www.cdc.gov

National Heart, Lung, and Blood Institute
www.nhlbi.nih.gov

National Institute of Diabetes and Digestive and Kidney Diseases (NIDDK)
www.niddk.nih.gov

National Institutes of Health
www.nih.gov

U.S. Department of Agriculture (USDA)
www.usda.gov

U.S. Department of Health and Human Services
www.dhhs.gov

U.S. Food and Drug Administration (FDA)
www.fda.gov

Smoking Cessation Resources

American Cancer Society
www.cancer.org/docroot/PED/content/PED_10_13X_Guide_for_Quitting_Smoking.asp

CDC Office on Smoking and Health
www.cdc.gov/tobacco

Smokefree.gov
http://smokefree.gov

Stop Smoking Foundation
www.stopsmoking.net

Food and Nutrition Resources

American Dietetic Association
www.eatright.org

Food and Nutrition Information Center
www.nal.usda.gov/fnic

Organic Food Resources

Horizon Organic Dairy
www.horizondairy.com

The National Directory of Farmers Markets
www.ams.usda.gov/AMSv1.0/FarmersMarkets

Organic.org
http://organic.org

Organicfood.net
http://organicfood.net

Organic Trade Association
www.ota.com

USDA Agricultural Marketing Service
www.ams.usda.gov

Natural Food Chains

Trader Joe's
www.traderjoes.com

Whole Foods Market, Inc.
www.wholefoods.com

Obesity Resources

Centers For Disease Control and Prevention Obesity
www.cdc.gov/obesity

The Obesity Society
www.obesity.org

Weight-Control Information Network
www.niddk.nih.gov/health/nutrit/pubs/health.htm

World Health Organization Obesity
www.who.int/topics/obesity/en

Exercise Resources

Aerobics and Fitness Association of America (AFAA)
www.afaa.com

American College of Sports Medicine
www.acsm.org

American Council on Exercise
www.acefitness.org

American Senior Fitness Association
www.seniorfitness.net

Aquatic Exercise Association (AEA)
www.aeawave.com

Disabled Sports Organizations
www.dsusa.org

International Council on Active Aging
www.icaa.cc

Medical Fitness Association (MFA)
www.medicalfitness.org

The National Center on Physical Activity and Disability
www.ncpad.org

Department of Disability and Human Development University of Illinois at Chicago
www.ahs.uic.edu/dhd

National Strength and Conditioning Association
http://nsca-lift.org

President's Council on Fitness, Sports & Nutrition
www.fitness.gov

YMCA of the USA
www.ymca.net

Stress and Wellness Resources

American Institute of Stress
www.stress.org

Learning Meditation
www.learningmeditation.com

Mayo Clinic Relaxation Techniques
www.mayoclinic.com/health/relaxation-technique/SR00007

The Meditation Society of America
www.meditationsociety.com

WebMD Stress Management Health Center
www.webmd.com/balance/stress-management/default.htm

Calculating Your Body Mass Index

The body mass index (BMI) is a measure that reduces the relationship between weight and height to one number. When you compare your BMI value to charted ranges, you get an approximation of body fatness, rather than a precise measure. The figure is not equal to a measurement of body-fat percentage.

The value of knowing your BMI is that it provides a rough estimate of whether your body size indicates a need to manage your weight more effectively.

To find your BMI, use the formula below, or check the Body Mass Index Chart for an approximate value. To understand what your BMI means, check the BMI categories for men and women. Overweight is defined as a BMI of 25–29.9; obesity is defined as a BMI equal to or more than 30. These numbers may not apply to pregnant women or muscular athletes.

Calculate Your BMI

The BMI was created using the metric system. To calculate your BMI, you can take your weight in kilograms and divide it by the square (a number multiplied by itself) of your height in meters. If you are more likely using pounds and inches, follow this simple three-step method:

1. Multiply your weight by 703.
2. Divide the result by your height.
3. Divide the result again by your height to get your BMI.

For example: If you are five foot seven (or 67" tall) and weigh 170 pounds, you would do the following:

1. Multiply $170 \times 703 = 119,510$.
2. Divide 119,510 by 67 = 1,785.
3. Divide 1,785 by 67 = 26.6.

In this example, the BMI is 26.6; this BMI falls in the overweight category.

Body Mass Index Chart

For a less precise answer without the math, here is a chart for men and women that gives the body mass index (BMI) for various heights (in inches) and weights (in pounds, with underwear but no shoes). Find your height, read across the row to your weight, then read up the column to find your approximate BMI score.

▼ THE BODY MASS INDEX CHART

BMI Score	21	22	23	24	25	26	27	28	29	30	31
4'10"	100	105	110	115	119	124	129	134	138	143	148
5'0"	107	112	118	123	128	133	138	143	148	153	158
5'1"	111	116	122	127	132	137	143	148	153	158	164
5'3"	118	124	130	135	141	146	152	158	163	169	175
5'5"	126	132	138	144	150	156	162	168	174	180	186
5'7"	134	140	146	153	159	166	172	178	185	191	198
5'9"	142	149	155	162	169	176	182	189	196	203	209
6'0"	150	157	165	172	179	186	193	200	208	215	222
6'1"	159	166	174	182	189	197	204	212	219	227	235
6'3"	168	176	184	192	200	208	216	224	232	240	248

What Does Your BMI Mean?

BMI ranges from 18.5–24.9.
Normal weight: Good for you! Try not to gain weight.

BMI ranges from 25–29.9.
Overweight: Try not to gain weight, especially if your waist measurement is high. You need to manage your weight if you have two or more risk factors for heart disease and are overweight, or have a high waist measurement.

BMI is 30 or greater.
Obese: You need to manage your weight. Lose weight slowly—about ½–2 pounds a week. See your doctor or a registered dietitian if you need help.

Source: *Clinical Guidelines on the Identification, Evaluation, and Treatment of Overweight and Obesity in Adults*; National Heart, Lung, and Blood Institute, in cooperation with the National Institute of Diabetes and Digestive and Kidney Diseases, National Institutes of Health, June 1998.

Index

We Have

EVERYTHING®

on Anything!

The Everything® list spans a wide range of subjects, with more than 500 titles covering 25 different categories:

Business	History	Reference
Careers	Home Improvement	Religion
Children's Storybooks	Everything Kids	Self-Help
Computers	Languages	Sports & Fitness
Cooking	Music	Travel
Crafts and Hobbies	New Age	Wedding
Education/Schools	Parenting	Writing
Games and Puzzles	Personal Finance	
Health	Pets	